UNDERGROUND CURES

THE MOST URGENT HEALTH SECRETS

E D I T I O N **IV**

680CB0002

Underground Cures: The Most Urgent Health Secrets. Edition IV
Published by Agora Health Books
Alice Jacob, Managing Editor
Ken Danz, Copy Editor

ISBN 1-891434-15-2
Printed in the United States of America

Agora Health Books
819 N. Charles Street
Baltimore, MD 21201
www.agorahealthbooks.com

UNDERGROUND CURES

THE MOST URGENT HEALTH SECRETS

E D I T I O N IV

Agora Health Books
Baltimore, Maryland

DISCLAIMER

All material in this publication is provided for information only and may not be construed as medical advice or instruction. No action should be taken based solely on the contents of this publication; instead, readers should consult appropriate health professionals on any matter relating to their health and well-being.

Nothing noted in the text should be considered an attempt by the publisher to practice medicine, prescribe remedies, make diagnoses, or act as persuasion for enforcing some mode of treatment, therapy, or surgery. The information and opinions provided in this publication are believed to be accurate and sound, based on the best judgment available to the authors, but readers who fail to consult with appropriate health authorities assume the risk of any injuries. The publisher is not responsible for errors or omissions.

THE INFORMATION PRESENTED HERE HAS NOT BEEN EVALUATED BY THE U.S. FOOD & DRUG ADMINISTRATION. THIS PRODUCT IS NOT INTENDED TO DIAGNOSE, TREAT, CURE, OR PREVENT ANY DISEASE.

Table of Contents

Introduction

Agora Health Books first teamed up with the Health Sciences Institute (HSI) five years ago to bring you the first edition of *Underground Cures*, a compilation of the most urgent health discoveries and groundbreaking research coming out of the world's top progressive clinics and research laboratories. We have once again partnered with HSI in the creation of the fourth edition of *Underground Cures* featuring the latest breakthrough healing solutions. These up-to-the minute discoveries will not only have you leaps and bounds ahead of the mainstream medical establishment, but you will find that in many cases you are steps ahead of even the alternative medical community.

We have filled this brand new edition of *Underground Cures* with 31 new chapters containing secrets for enhancing your health, extending your life, and liberating yourself from the devastating effects of many serious conditions. With categories ranging from cancer to diabetes and from immunity building to pain relief *Underground Cures* is destined to become a permanent reference book in your home library.

Every day, around the world, researchers and scientists are making exciting medical breakthroughs and health discoveries. Yet, you are often deprived of these healing possibilities. Your doctor may simply be too busy to sift through all the latest research. Or maybe he is overly influenced by the big pharmaceutical companies. Or perhaps a potentially lifesaving treatment is trapped in the tangles of government bureaucracy. The bottom line is this...for one reason or another you are not getting the health information you need when you need it.

In 1996, a small, private group of conventionally and holistically trained doctors formed a network through which they could rapidly exchange news of the latest, most innovative cures and overcome bureaucratic blocks and delays.

This network is the Health Sciences Institute, dedicated to uncovering and researching the most urgent advances in modern underground medicine, like those you will read about in this book. The hard work and commitment of these "underground" health pioneers brings these cures to light...so that you can use them today.

The Health Sciences Institute now has over 85,000 members worldwide. As it grows in international reputation, more laboratories and scientists send news of their research directly to the institute. The editors at HSI research the truly revolutionary breakthroughs for safety, efficacy, and availability.

Every day, stacks of letters arrive from people whose lives were changed by a breakthrough they learned of through the HSI network. The institute maintains a file of members who have overcome such diseases as arthritis, prostate disorders, fatigue, and depression...of members who, although they had nearly given up hope, experienced dramatic recoveries when they tried a remedy they read about in an HSI publication. For information on how to become a member of the Health Sciences Institute and receive regular news of the latest medical breakthroughs please turn to page 223.

Breakthroughs
In Conquering Cancer

Cancer is deceptively easy to define. It is a group of diseases that are characterized by an uncontrolled growth and spread of abnormal cells. But anyone who has been faced with cancer—either through fighting it themselves or through watching a loved one fight it—knows that it is far more difficult to understand than this simple definition implies.

The statistics are downright frightening. According to the American Cancer Society in 2003 alone 1,334,100 new cancer cases are expected to be diagnosed and 556,500 cancer deaths are expected to occur. That is a mind-boggling 1,500 people a day! In fact cancer is the second leading cause of death in the United States; second only to heart disease. With 1 out of 4 of us dying at the hands of this killer the word cancer has even become synonymous with the concept of a spreading evil.

But the good news reveals itself when you take a closer look at the statistics. The **majority** of people diagnosed with cancer **are** going to survive it. In fact the experts estimate that there are around 8.9 million cancer survivors living in America alone! And with regular screenings and continued education about lifestyle changes this number is expected to keep rising. With conventional and alternative prevention techniques and treatments working hand in hand more and more of us are expected to defeat this killer—or even avoid it altogether.

In this section you will find the results of up-to-the-minute breakthroughs in cancer prevention and treatment techniques. You will read about the exciting research that has revealed that a small tree that grows in the wild in the Amazon—and that has long been used in the herbal traditions of the local people—packs a potent cancer-fighting punch. You will learn about the immunity-boosting medicinal mushroom that many give credit to for the good health and longevity of a small community in Brazil. You'll find a chapter on a cream that might be the key to eliminating pre-cancerous skin lesions, one on the seaweed cancer treatment that is a staple in the diet of many in one long-lived Japanese community, another on the powerful phytocompounds that have gained the attention of a major biotech company, and finally one on a natural sunscreen that offers a nearly-perfect defense against the damaging rays of the sun.

Agaricus Blazei Murrill (ABM) Mushroom:
Discover the cancer-fighting potential of Brazil's "Mushroom of God"

Nearly 30 years ago researchers began investigating a medical curiosity among the people of Piedade, Brazil. Residents of the small community near Sao Paulo enjoyed extraordinarily good health. They developed few diseases and lived unusually long lives. Outsiders began to wonder what was enhancing the Brazilians' immunity and lifespan. In their quest for an answer, researchers stumbled upon the "Mushroom of God."

Depending on which account you believe, it was either two researchers from Penn State or Taktoshi Furumoto, a Japanese farmer living in Brazil, who solved the puzzle. He (or they) zeroed in on a small, wild mushroom that locals ate regularly, believing it fostered good health. It was commonly known as Cogumelo de Deus or Cogumelo do Sol—Mushroom of God or Mushroom of the Sun.

Regardless of who discovered it, it was Japanese researchers (doctors from Tokyo University and Japan's National Cancer Center, in particular) who eventually subjected the mushroom to pharmacological testing. They reported that the mushroom, which eventually acquired the botanical name *Agaricus Blazei Murill* (ABM), could be a potent immune-builder and cancer-fighter.

To date, ABM has not been used in any human clinical trials. All research has been performed in petri dishes or laboratory animals. However, news of this rare medicinal mushroom has already prompted between 300,000 and 500,000 Japanese people to supplement with ABM, hoping to prevent cancer or stop the disease from recurring. Numerous others consume it regularly reportedly to avoid infection, diabetes, hyperlipidemia, chronic hepatitis, and arteriosclerosis.

ABM enhances the immune response to protect you from cancer

In recent years, Japanese research has confirmed that ABM contains a host of health-promoting components: vitamins B_1 and B_2, niacin, phosphorous, iron, calcium, protein, amino acids, and ergosterol (which converts into vitamin D_2 when the mushroom is dried). But most importantly, the researchers discovered that ABM contains large quantities of active polysaccharides—complex carbohydrates, most commonly found in foods like wheat, rice, and potatoes that stimulate the immune system to fight off bacterial and viral illnesses.[1]

ABM stimulates the immune system by triggering the production of:

- T-cells, which directly attack cells that have been taken over by viruses or cancers[2];

- interleukin, which bolsters the immune system by stimulating the growth and activity of white blood cells;

- tumor necrosis factor (TNF), which activates white blood cells and fights tumors;

- and macrophages, which protect the body from infection by consuming foreign material.[3]

Obviously, a list of in vitro and animal studies (with no human trials in the mix) is not proof that ABM is an effective cancer treatment. Products, whether they are natural or pharmaceutical, need to pass more extensive and rigorous testing to support such a claim.

In several studies, however, ABM has stimulated animals' immune systems and arrested the growth of their tumors. And in the past, HSI has documented the ability of other medicinal mushrooms, such as AHCC, to build immunity and help people fight cancer (see the *HSI Members Alert* issues for January 2000 and January 2002 or search online at www.HSIBaltimore.com). We don't know yet if ABM will eventually rank with those health-promoting mushrooms. But the preliminary evidence was compelling enough that we decided to analyze it and report the findings to you.

Retard tumor growth by 90 percent in just three weeks

At Japan's Ehime University School of Medicine, researchers tested ABM's impact on tumors. Twenty days of treatment with certain ABM extracts (800 mg/kg per day taken orally) retarded tumor growth in cancerous mice between 80 and 90 percent. The researchers determined that the tumor-retarding agent was ergosterol, a steroid alcohol that occurs naturally in mold and yeast.

So they conducted a second experiment, giving oral doses of ergosterol (between 100 and 800 mg/kg) daily to tumor-bearing mice for 20 days. The treatment "significantly reduced tumor growth" in a dose-dependent manner. Mice given the largest doses experienced 85.5 percent less tumor growth than mice treated with placebos. The ergosterol, however, did not destroy cancer cells directly. Instead, it inhibited the development of new blood vessels within the tumor—a process that can stop and eventually reverse tumor growth. The treatment also produced another benefit: After 20 days of treatment none of the mice were suffering any of the side effects typically induced by chemotherapy drugs.[4]

Using guinea pigs as guinea pigs

Cancerous guinea pigs experienced even greater recovery rates—over 99 percent—when they were treated with ABM. Researchers from Tokyo College of Pharmacy, Tokyo University, and Japan's National Cancer Center Laboratory injected cancer cells into the femur (thighbone) of each pig—a procedure that normally causes cancer to spread throughout the animal's body within four to five weeks.

Twenty-four hours later (once the cancer cells were embedded in the animals' tissue), the researchers gave the pigs ABM injections and continued to give them daily injections for 10 consecutive days. Five weeks later, 99.4 percent of the guinea pigs had fully recovered from the cancer.[5]

Other scientists tested ABM's ability to fight cancer by first injecting tumor cells in both the right and left flanks of laboratory mice. The scientists then injected ABM fractions into the mice, but only into their right-flank tumors. The injections inhibited tumor growth in the right flank, and even caused regression in some cases. But the treatment also inhibited growth of left-flank tumors. The researchers who were based at Japan's Miyagi Cancer Center Research Institute, speculated that the ABM had triggered the immune system to unleash more white blood cells to all cancerous areas, not just those specifically injected with the extract.[6]

Granted, that's a lot of speculation. And all of these trials may make you want to give thanks you're not a rodent living anywhere near a Japanese laboratory. But the dramatic results shown by the mice and guinea pigs tested certainly seem reason enough to investigate ABM further to determine if it's anywhere near as promising for us humans with cancer.

Extreme growing conditions make mushroom a rare commodity

Unfortunately, accessing supplies of ABM mushrooms or ABM supplements has been difficult. For decades, growers were unable to successfully cultivate this wild mushroom. It typically thrives in extreme conditions—intense Brazilian sunlight, humidity averaging 80 percent, and temperatures that soar to 100 degrees during the day and drop to 68 degrees overnight. It was only in the early '90s that growers devised a method of producing biologically active ABM mushrooms in beds of pasteurized horse manure and sugar cane residue (hardly appetizing, but reportedly it creates a powerful growing medium).

Today, Japanese consumers purchase 90 percent of Brazil's yearly ABM crop. Consequently, you're not likely to find fresh ABM mushrooms in even the best produce markets in America.

A few supplement companies, however, have begun producing ABM tablets (which are already hot sellers in Japan). No clinical trials have yet been published about these supplements. (All the published trials involve ABM extracts. The supplements typically contain whole mushrooms that have been freeze-dried and powdered.) So, the exact impact of ABM supplementation isn't known. But, again, our experience with other similar supplements makes us less skeptical.

If you try ABM, let us know about your experience with it. HSI will continue to search for information on this promising mushroom and for a source for the extract. For ordering information see the Source Directory on page 213.

COULD THIS BRAZILIAN MUSHROOM
HOLD THE SECRET TO BETTER CHEMO?

If ABM shows such promise on its own for fighting cancer, it seems logical to assume that it could enhance the effects of conventional cancer treatments. But when it comes to your health, assuming isn't nearly enough.

At Mie University in Japan, researchers conducted a series of tests with ABM and the cancer chemotherapy drug, 5-fluorouracil (5-FU). Administered alone (at a dosage of 10mg/kg for 30 days), the ABM extract moderately inhibited tumor growth in cancerous mice. Treatment with both ABM and 5-FU strongly inhibited tumor growth in the mice.

The more interesting results, however, centered around ABM's effects on 5-FU. First, it prolonged the action of 5-FU, which, like many chemotherapy drugs, is only effective on its own for a short period of time. Second, it offset the drastic immune-system weakening usually caused by chemotherapy. At the end of the experiment, mice treated with the ABM/5-FU combination showed "significantly increased" numbers of immune-modulating cells compared to the mice treated with saline only.[7]

References

[1] Agricultural and Biological Chemistry, 54(11): 2897-2906, 1990

[2] Biosci Biotechnol Biochem, 62(3): 434, 1998 Mar

[3] Cell Struct Funct, 26(2): 103-8, 2001 Apr

[4] J Nutr, 131(5): 1,409-13, 2001 May

[5] www.shikoku.ne.jp

[6] Biotherapy, 11(4): 259-65, 1998

[7] Jpn J Pharmacol, 66(2): 265-71, 1994 Oct

Glycoalkaloid cream:
Cream eliminates 83 percent of pre-cancerous lesions in small-scale trial

Sometimes our efforts to seek out and report leading-edge developments in alternative health care hit startling roadblocks.

Take, for example, our plan to bring you a product update on glycoalkaloid cream. It seemed simple enough. The product, which we first told you about in 1998, had proven effective in easing a common—and menacing—age-related condition in both research experiments and clinical use.

So we were stunned when the formulator—a reputable, scientifically oriented company with a long history in alternative healthcare—called and begged us to drop its name from the story. Just a few days earlier, the Food and Drug Administration (FDA) contacted the company and warned that it could be the subject of government action if it made any claims that its products treat disease.

You see, FDA regulations stipulate that only FDA-approved products can make claims about fighting or treating disease. And natural products rarely get approved by the FDA. Formulators of botanicals and natural medicines generally can't afford to seek FDA approval (pharmaceutical companies spend an average of $300-600 million bringing each drug to market) simply because they can't patent a natural substance and recoup their investment.

Consequently, even if a dozen clinical trials conclude that a Japanese mushroom formulation shrinks tumors, the formulator can never broadcast that claim. Sometimes, even disease statements in the press, which is still protected by the First Amendment as far as we know, appear risky for supplement formulators.

So, at the request of the manufacturer, who is under pressure from the FDA, we won't publish the following information as an official product update. But we have a responsibility to you to report this sort of important information as we receive it. So we will refer to the product simply as glycoalkaloid cream—a natural formulation that may help you repair sun-damaged skin and avoid a battle with cancer.

Eliminating "age spots" may reduce your risk of skin cancer

More than half of us over age 50 have them—raised rough, scaly brown spots or red spots on our faces, necks, limbs, and shoulders. They're called seborhheic keratosis and gradually roughen to become actinic keratoses (AKs). At best, they're the less-than-desirable marks created by too much time in the sun. At worst, they're the preliminary stages of skin cancer.

Skin cancer will afflict 1.3 million Americans this year and kill roughly 2,200. AKs are the most common form of premalignant lesions. If left untreated, they can evolve into squamous cell carcinoma and heighten your risk of developing malignant melanoma (a much more deadly form of skin cancer.) But that progression can be stopped.

In 1998, we first told readers about skin creams containing glycoalkaloids (chemical compounds extracted from the Australian "devil's apple") that could destroy AKs before they had a chance to degenerate into cancer. Now new research and recent clinical experience confirms that as little as one month of treatment with glycoalkaloids can eradicate AKs, relieving patients of skin blemishes, inflammation, and a risk of cancer.

Researchers at New York Presbyterian Hospital and Cornell Medical Center in New York recruited outpatients with AKs to test the effectiveness of the cream. It was a small trial—just six subjects. But the results were striking. Patients were instructed to apply the cream to their lesions twice a day for six weeks. Researchers examined the patients every two weeks and reported that the treatment completely eliminated the spots on 83.3 percent of patients. In two patients, the lesions disappeared within four weeks.[1]

The treatment triggered one side effect. Five of the six subjects reported experiencing mild to severe skin irritation, which lessened as the lesions disappeared. But this effect did not prompt any of the patients to discontinue treatment.[2]

Cream helps abnormal—even cancerous—skin return to normal in as little as one month

According to laboratory research, glycoalkaloids (also referred to as solasodine glycoside) selectively target precancerous and cancerous cells. They penetrate the weaker walls of these abnormal cells and trigger cell death.

An Australian study involving 72 patients reported that treatment with solasodine glycosides cream resulted in full regression of 100 percent of precancerous and cancerous conditions. Treatment took up to three months to become effective, and triggered severe skin irritation in some cases.[3]

Benefits reach beyond cancer, helping skin conditions like eczema, dermatitis, and psoriasis

Ross Hauser, M.D.—Medical Director of Caring Medical and Rehabilitation Services (a natural health clinic) in Oak Park, Illinois—has treated several hundred patients with glycoalkaloid cream. "It's very potent. If there is a pre-malignant lesion or sun-damaged area, it helps restore the skin to normal...usually within a month," he says.

Dr. Hauser recommends the cream to patients with all sorts of skin diseases and disorders, not just to those patients with pre-cancerous lesions. "A lot of times when a person has a skin problem, you don't even know what it is," he says. "I've done a lot of biopsies on skin lesions and [the results] almost always come back as non-descript inflammation." Conventional treatment for this sort of general inflammation generally involves using a steroidal cream, which can actually weaken the skin. Some natural medicine practitioners even argue that steroidal creams can drive a surface disease deeper into the body.

Alternative medicine includes numerous treatments for skin diseases. However given the often ambiguous nature of skin disease, Dr. Hauser typically recommends patients try a glycoalkaloid cream instead. "There's a danger in using calendula cream or some other homeopathic treatment that doesn't have the ability to treat a pre-cancerous lesion and make it normal skin. You don't want to just treat [the lesion] with some kind of herbal combination and then find out you've got some dangerous skin lesion, some kind of skin cancer."

According to Dr. Hauser, glycoalkaloid cream has effectively treated eczema, allergic dermatitis, and some cases of psoriasis among his patients.

For information on ordering glycoalkaloid cream see the Source Directory starting on page 213.

IS IT A MOLE—OR IS IT CANCER?

Cosmetics commercials call them "signs of aging." As we get older, most of us develop more spots on our skin. Most are benign little nuisances. But some can be the first signs of skin cancer.

Actinic keratosis is literally an overgrowth of tissue caused by chemical changes in the skin. Those chemical changes are triggered by exposure to radiant energy, such as ultraviolet light.

Unlike a simple mole, AKs are irregularly shaped patches of raised, rough, scaly skin that's deep red or brown. You'll find them most often on the exposed skin of middle-aged and elderly individuals with fair complexions. AKs can also develop as a roughening and whitening of common flat, brown pigmented "age" or "liver" spots. Cancer specialists will urge you to conduct monthly self-examinations for spots of sun-damaged skin.

Conventional treatment for AKs typically involves either cryosurgery using liquid nitrogen or a topical treatment of Efudex® (a cream containing the cancer drug 5-fluorouracil which can produce severe side effects).

References

[1] "Efficacy of solasodine cream for treatment of actinic keratoses," Dr. Babar Rao, et al

[2] ibid.

[3] Cancer Lett 1991 Sept; 59(3): 183-92

CHAPTER 3

Fucoidan:
Cancer's kryptonite: HSI panelist tests breakthrough seaweed cancer treatment

with commentary by Kohhei Makise, M.D.

It's a weed and a slimy weed at that. But unlike the ones that invade your lawn, this weed might actually do you some good. It has been credited as a primary cause for record-low cancer rates in Okinawa, Japan. It was used—with reported success—to treat and prevent radiation sickness following the Chernobyl meltdown in Russia. It has yet to be tested in a single human clinical trial. But according to panelist Kohhei Makise, M.D., the Japanese medical community is being inundated with reports of how this medicinal seaweed has helped thousands of patients fight cancer.

Dr. Makise recently wrote us a long, excited e-mail discussing several new natural remedies that are producing impressive results among Japanese patients. (And yes, we will share more of Dr. Makise's insights in upcoming Health Sciences Institute issues. For information on joining HSI please see page 223.) But for now, we decided to focus on a natural immune builder and cancer fighter that's so new to North America that we'd never heard of it before.

It's called fucoidan, and it's a complex of polysaccharides (carbohydrates) found in brown seaweed, most commonly in an Asia-Pacific variety known as *kombu* or *Laminaria japonica*. The seaweed has been a dietary staple in Japan since the second century B.C. And in Okinawa—which posts Japan's highest per capita rates of *kombu* consumption—it has reportedly produced considerable health benefits. Okinawa residents who eat an average of 1 gram of *kombu* (containing roughly 5 mg of fucoidan) daily enjoy some of the longest lifespans in Japan and the single lowest cancer rate in the country.

Seaweed extract causes cancer cells to self-destruct

In the 1990s, scientists identified fucoidan as the primary immune-building substance in brown seaweed and began to test it.

In one case, researchers injected female lab rats with a carcinogen known to induce mammary tumors. They fed half of the rats a standard diet, fed the other half a standard diet plus daily helpings of brown seaweed containing fucoidan, and monitored the animals for 26 weeks. The fucoidan appeared to convey two substantial benefits. First, the fucoidan-fed rats developed fewer tumors than the control rats: 63 percent developed breast cancer vs. 76 percent of control rats. Second, the fucoidan-fed rats resisted developing tumors for longer periods of time: control rats typically developed tumors within 11 weeks, whereas fucoidan-fed rats remained cancer-free for 19 weeks.[1]

In other studies, oral and intravenous doses of brown seaweed proved anywhere from 61.9 to 95.2 percent effective in preventing the development of cancer in rats implanted with sarcoma cells.[2] One group of researchers described fucoidan as a "very potent anti-tumor agent in cancer therapy" after it inhibited the growth and spread of lung cancer in rats.[3] (That type of cancer is particularly resistant to chemotherapy.)

Various studies further demonstrated that fucoidan combats cancer in multiple ways:

- It causes certain types of rapidly growing cancer cells (including stomach cancer, colon cancer, and leukemia) to self-destruct (a process call apoptosis).

- It physically interferes with cancer cells' ability to adhere to tissue. That interference prevents the cancer from spreading (or metastasizing) to new areas.

- It enhances production of several immune mechanisms, including macrophages (white blood cells that destroy tumor cells), gamma interferon (proteins that activate macrophages and natural killer cells), and interleukin (compounds that help regulate the immune system).

Proof from the panelist's practice

But as Dr. Makise points out, fucoidan still needs to prove itself in large, double-blind, clinical trials involving creatures more evolved than guinea pigs. (To date, all the testing of fucoidan has been conducted in petri dishes or on small laboratory animals.)

Dr. Makise believes, however, that there is compelling evidence that fucoidan can help prevent cancer. Through his practice in Japan, Dr. Makise has seen that fucoidan can even help patients who already have cancer. He says that cancer patients benefit most by taking a combination of:

- fucoidan
- AHCC or other immune enhancing mushrooms
- antioxidants, especially large doses of selenium
- enterococcus feacalis—1 to 3 trillion dead bacterium (Enterococcus faecalis is a beneficial bacterial found in the intestine. In addition to promoting healthy digestion and controlling bile acids that can cause colon cancer, it delivers certain immune-enhancing vitamins—like biotin and certain B vitamins—to the blood stream)
- essential daily vitamins and minerals (Dr. Makise recommends his patients take triple the recommended daily dosage of essential vitamins and minerals. He says it's especially important that cancer patients take daily supplements of selenium and zinc)
- a healthy lifestyle and diet that avoids meat, milk and other animal proteins and fats.

"It is very effective for cancers that already exist, even end-stage metastases," Dr. Makise told us. "Each substance of this combination has a different mechanism to fight against cancer, so we get synergistic effects.

"Of course this combination is never a panacea. It can never save the lives of 100 percent of cancer patients. But my impression is that 30 to 40 percent of cancer patients are much improved on this combination." According to Dr. Makise, even some terminal patients have benefited from the regimen, experiencing less pain and a better quality of life in their final months.

The fine print on fucoidan-based therapy

This treatment regimen, Dr. Makise concedes, has two problems. First, it's expensive. The roster of supplements can easily cost $500 a month and, unfortunately, isn't covered by medical insurance plans in Japan or the United States. Second, no single cancer therapy—conventional or alternative—works for each patient or every cancer. Consequently, finding the exact supplement mixture and dosage that will work for each individual is tricky. Dr. Makise tracks his patients' immune function (by measuring interleukin levels, natural killer cell counts, etc.) to determine how to adjust their supplements. "If we find the immune system of the patient gets low, we increase the dose of the supplements or change the supplements or add other supplements such as organic germanium, shark cartilage, etc. But we find the combination is generally much safer, much more gentle, and definitely more effective than chemotherapy alone, except for cases of leukemia and malignant lymphoma."

The fucoidan challenge:
Getting your hands on this seaweed miracle

It's an occupational hazard that we're trying to turn into an opportunity. When your job is to research leading-edge developments in alternative health care around the globe, you inevitably stumble across remedies that are being widely used with impressive results in some distant nation, but flat out aren't available in North America.

That's the dilemma we ran into when we started researching fucoidan. Dr. Makise has seen many cancer patients get considerable benefit from one fucoidan product. But the Japanese corporation that manufactured that product didn't export to the United States and, for its own business reasons, didn't want to start.

So we've been searching for alternatives. We asked Dr. Makise to analyze the one fucoidan supplement that is available in the U.S. He warned us that the product contained a substance (iodine) that would make it inappropriate for some patients, and that the product had a sufficiently different chemical makeup that he couldn't be sure it would generate the same kinds of benefits his patients had experienced.

So we went back to our search, started flipping through our list of contacts, and got in touch with the president of American BioSciences, the company that brought AHCC to North America. We knew American

---

A NEW ERA OF CANCER TREATMENT: FUCOIDAN COMPLEMENTS TRADITION WHILE STARTING ITS OWN

Perhaps one of the most intriguing aspects of fucoidan is that not only does it work well in its own right to fight cancer, but it can also help patients undergoing chemotherapy achieve greater results.

Researchers at Mie University in Japan actually documented the ability of fucoidan to enhance the action of the chemotherapy drug 5FU. They removed primary Lewis lung carcinoma (LLC) tumors from lab rats, then tracked the ability of different treatments to prevent the metastasis often caused by LLC. (Lung cancer patients often develop secondary cancers even though the primary tumor has been surgically removed.) Fucoidan "significantly inhibited" metastasis when given alone or in conjunction with 5FU.

At the end of the study, they discovered that the lungs of animals given fucoidan contained more macrophages than other animals. And macrophages are key to fighting cancer by destroying tumor cells and stimulating other components of the immune system. The fucoidan also directly helped the 5FU fight cancer. Animals given fucoidan retained higher concentrations of 5FU in lung tissue, liver, blood, kidneys and spleen than animals given drug treatment only. The fucoidan also helped the drug remain active longer.[4]

So even if you prefer a more conventional approach to cancer treatment, you may want to consider adding fucoidan to your regimen to ensure you get as much benefit as possible from whatever therapy you choose.

BioSciences had developed extensive contacts within the Japanese supplement industry. And as luck would have it, the president had recently started researching seaweed extracts. We put him in touch with Dr. Makise, and sent them both off to find us an acceptable and available fucoidan product.

For information on ordering fucoidan see the Source Directory starting on page 213.

References

[1] Cell Bio Toxicol, 13 (2): 95-102, 1997 Feb

[2] Radiats Biol Radioecol, 39(5): 572-7, 1999 Sep-Oct

[3] Eur J Haematol, 54 (1): 27-33, 1995 Jan

[4] Anticancer Res, 15(5B): 1,937-47, 1995 Sep-Oct

Guacatonga:

Get access to the latest breakthrough in cancer research–even before the drug companies

Maybe you've heard of Taxol®. It's a prescription drug used to fight cancer, particularly cancer of the ovary, breast, and lung.

But what you might *not* know is that Taxol is derived from a plant source: the bark of the Pacific yew tree. Researchers first identified the bark's anti-tumor potential in 1963—and then it took the pharmaceutical industry nearly *30 years* to bring Taxol to market.

Now, we've learned that the same forces that developed Taxol are on the trail of a new novel cancer-fighter. That's good news for cancer patients—but it gets even better. We've got a direct route to the natural source, so you don't have to wait a decade or more while the drug companies wade through red tape. And, through a special arrangement, we can make this promising new anticancer therapy available *right now* to those who need it most.

Research shows plant from the Amazon can fight cancer

Casearia sylvestris is the Latin name for a small tree that grows in the wilds of the Amazon. It's been known by a variety of other names in various cultures, but it's perhaps best known by the name *guacatonga*. The bark, leaves, and roots of this tree have long been part of the herbal medicine traditions in the lands where it grows. But it's the leaves and twigs that have caught the attention of some of the mainstream's heavy hitters—groups like the National Cancer Institute, Research Triangle Institute (the group that uncovered the power of the Pacific yew), and Bristol-Myers Squibb (the pharmaceutical company that produces Taxol).

The February 2002 issue of the *Journal of Natural Products* includes a study funded by an NCI grant and administered by scientists from RTI and Bristol-Myers Squibb, along with researchers from the University of Illinois at Chicago and a university in Ecuador. The study identifies "three novel clerodane diterpenoids" in guacatonga that show "promising bioactivity," particularly in tests against a variety of tumor cell lines.[1]

The science behind guacatonga is quite complex, and so is the trail of research on the plant that spans nearly 20 years. Like this new study, most of it focuses on *clerodane diterpenoids*, a class of hydrocarbon compounds found in many types of plants.

A group of scientists at the Tokyo College of Pharmacy were actually the first to find the clerodane diterpenoids in guacatonga. In 1988, these researchers identified three unique *clerodane diterpenoids* in the plant, which they labeled *casearins A, B,* and *C.* Then they conducted a series of animal trials to assess the efficacy of these casearins against cancer. They tested an ethanol-based casearin extract against sarcoma and various other

---

MORE PIECES IN GUACATONGA'S HEALING PUZZLE

While research into guacatonga's anticancer benefits lay dormant, scientists continued to study the plant's other medicinal uses. And they found compelling evidence to support guacatonga's healing power in a number of areas.

In traditional herbal medicine, guacatonga has long been a remedy for stomach ailments and ulcers. Now modern science supports that claim. In a Brazilian trial, researchers found that guacatonga extract was as effective as several prescription drugs in preventing stress-induced stomach ulcers in laboratory mice. They determined that guacatonga protected against ulcers by inhibiting gastric secretions and reducing hydrochloric acid output.[5]

Guacatonga is also traditionally used to treat bites from poisonous snakes and insects—a common problem in the rainforests of the Amazon. Researchers have found significant evidence to support this application. Scientists at the Universidade Federal de

---

human cancer cell lines. And in all cases, they reported that the guacatonga showed promising cytotoxic and anti-tumor activity.[2] In fact, the scientists were so encouraged by their findings that they filed a Japanese patent on the three clerodane diterpenoids they found in the plant.

For some unknown reason, the Japanese scientists never pursued their patent. But because it remained in place, other research groups were reluctant to pursue further study on guacatonga—until now. The RTI research identified three new clerodane diterpenoids, which they labeled *casearvestrins A, B,* and *C.* And the effects of these three newly discovered compounds were quite impressive. All showed cytotoxic effects against lung, colon, mouth, and ovarian cancer cells in laboratory tests, when compared to controls.[3]

There are still many unanswered questions about exactly *how* the phytochemicals in this rainforest plant fight cancer. Some studies have suggested

---

MORE PIECES IN GUACATONGA'S HEALING PUZZLE...*CONTINUED*

Uberlandia in Brazil, found that guacatonga extract significantly inhibits phosolipase A2 (PLA2), an enzyme that is widely distributed in venoms. In laboratory tests, guacatonga effectively inhibited the anticoagulant activity of PLA2 and partially reduced the swelling associated with snake bites.[6]

Phospholipase plays many roles in the body, and guacatonga's ability to inhibit this enzyme may explain many of its beneficial effects. For example, PLA2 is also present in digestive pancreatic secretions—a possible link to guacatonga's benefits in combatting stomach ulcers. Another type of PLA2 (known as PLA2 Type II) is thought to play a role in the genesis of inflammation, and another type of phospholopase, Type C, is a highly toxic secretion of some disease-causing bacteria.

Although researchers don't understand how all the pieces fit together, it's clear that guacatonga contains some powerful phytochemicals.

that the clerodane diterpenoids in the plant may kill cancer cells by damaging their DNA.[4] Another study found that the leaves and twigs of guacatonga contain another phytochemical called *lapachol*, the active ingredient in yet another Amazonian anticancer plant called *pau d'arco*.

New trial gives direct access to guacatonga right NOW

All this is very interesting…but how can it help you? Even with promising results like these, we're years away from seeing RTI and Bristol-Myers Squibb translate this information into treatment. After all, it took them almost 30 years to develop Taxol.

But if you're fighting cancer *now*, you don't have to wait. When HSI panelist Leslie Taylor learned about the work being done with guacatonga, she started doing some work of her own. She learned that the shamans of Indian medicine had been using the plant for centuries to treat all manner of ailments, including ulcers, inflammation, pain, and snake and insect bites. She learned that research by Brazilian scientists have found no evidence of any toxicity or side effects from the plant. *And* she located a source for guacatonga in its natural state, a source that can provide the plant's power right away.

Early imports available now

Raintree Nutrition, Inc., has just begun to import guacatonga and is offering it in capsule form. The product is showing very promising results and in fact Raintree is currently in the midst of conducting an observational study. Doctors from across the country have been recruited to participate in this informal trial of guacatonga on sarcoma patients. Remember, the original Japanese research back in 1988 showed that guacatonga was effective against sarcomas in laboratory mice. And sarcomas are some of the deadliest of all human cancers, so finding potential treatments for its victims is even more critical. Ms. Taylor has agreed to provide a free supply of guacatonga to these patients, and the doctors have agreed to track their progress over a 90-day course of treatment and supply the results to Raintree.

Tracking the trial results

We'll be keeping close tabs on the progress of the Raintree guacatonga trial, and we'll be sure to report the results in a future Health Sciences Institute newsletter and in the HSI e-Alert (see page 224 for information on how to sign up for the free HSI e-Alert) as soon as they are available. For more information on guacatonga see the Source Directory starting on page 213.

References
[1] Journal of Natural Products, ;65:95-99, 2002

[2] Chem Pharm Bull, 36:1585-1588, 1988

[3] Journal of Natural Products, 65:95-99, 2002

[4] An Acad Bras Cienc, 71:181-187, 1999

[5] J Ethnpharmacol, 30:185-197, 1990

[6] Comp Biochem Physiol B Biochem Mol Biol, 127:21-30, 2000

Larreastat™:
Sun protection straight from the Arizona desert

by Robert A. Sinnott, Ph.D.

By now, the media, with its incessant news reports, magazine articles, and general "public service" announcements, has drilled it into all of our heads that prolonged sun exposure leads to an increased risk of skin cancer. So we've followed the only advice we've been given: Stay out of the sun as much as possible, and when you do go out, cover up, wear a big floppy hat, and slather any exposed skin with sunscreen. Not exactly conducive to a carefree, fun-filled summer, but most of us figure it beats getting skin cancer.

However, very few people know why we've been told to take cover or what effect the sun actually has on our skin and other organs. And even fewer people know that there's an all-natural form of sunscreen—one that HSI reported on years ago in relation to its amazing effects on the herpes virus. I admit, skin cancer and herpes seem as completely unrelated as two health conditions could get. But you can find protection from both with the extract of a shrub that has been growing in the desert for centuries.

Are your skin cells on a sun-damage suicide mission?

Sunlight contains many different colors (or wavelengths) of light ranging from ultraviolet light to infrared light and all the visible colors in between. Most of those light waves are completely harmless since they cannot penetrate the outer layer of our skin. The real culprit is ultraviolet light, which is sufficiently energetic to penetrate deeply into our skin and damage the inner workings of cells. Specifically, it causes some fat molecules, which are present in all cells, to become free radicals—damaged molecules that can cause premature cell aging, genetic mutations in DNA, and even cell death.

If the genetic mutations are not too extensive, as with a mild sunburn, cells will attempt to repair themselves. However, if the mutations are extensive, such as in a severe sunburn, cells will initiate a suicide process rather than take the risk of becoming cancerous. When your skin peels several days after a sunburn, you know the damage to your DNA was too extensive for your body to repair, so the skin cells choose to commit suicide en masse. This system works remarkably well. Without it, we would all likely get skin cancer very early in our lives after only very brief sun exposure.

Of course, this system isn't 100 percent effective. Inevitably, some cells, badly damaged by sunlight, do not commit suicide. These mutated cells continue living in our skin and eventually may begin rapidly dividing and cause skin cancer.

Under attack:
The right message reaches the wrong cells

There is one other imperfection in the system. Sometimes the suicide message reaches other parts of your body besides the sunburned area of your skin. Cells of the immune system and cells infected with herpes viruses are especially likely to pick up this suicide signal. The herpes viruses read this suicide signal as saying, "The body is in trouble." But, rather than assisting your body, the herpes viruses sense your vulnerability and begin to attack. Dormant herpes viruses start replicating quickly in nerve cells and infected tissues. This is why outbreaks of cold sores, genital herpes or shingles (herpes zoster) may follow a period of prolonged sun exposure. Other less common diseases with a herpes virus component—multiple sclerosis, trigeminal neuralgia, herpetic neuralgia, Bell's palsy, Kaposi's sarcoma, and even Alzheimer's disease—can be aggravated by sun exposure.

So how do you protect yourself from these risks, short of becoming a recluse or buying stock in Coppertone?

The 100 percent natural sunscreen that has been growing in the desert for centuries

Not surprisingly, desert plants possess excellent defenses against damaging sun rays. Unlike animals that seek shade during the most intense periods of the day, plants must endure constant ultraviolet bombardment all day, every day. In Arizona—where some areas average 360 sunny days per year—that turns out to be a tremendous amount of sun exposure. Yet a shrub that is abundant in the Arizona desert—the *Larrea tridentata* or "creosote bush"—can live to be 12,000 years old. It protects itself by producing natural chemicals that function as both a sunscreen and an antioxidant. And evidence suggests those same chemicals can protect humans, too.

Larreastat is an extract from the leaves of the creostote bush, containing antiviral and anti-inflammatory agents. HSI members have known about Larreastat since it was first brought to market in 1996, and many have used it to successfully ease viral diseases (especially herpes viruses) and inflammatory disorders (including rheumatoid arthritis). It has been formulated into numerous products labeled as antioxidant dietary supplements and topical antioxidant cosmetics.

Larreastat can help protect people from ultraviolet skin damage in two distinct ways. First, the natural flavonoid compounds that make up approximately 50 percent of Larreastat's composition are violet-light absorbers, especially helpful in absorbing the light from the regions of the solar spectrum that are most likely to cause skin damage (the UV-A and UV-B regions). By absorbing light from these UV regions, Larreastat works as a traditional sunscreen—except that it is 100 percent natural.

The second way that Larreastat can protect from sun damage is that both major components in Larreastat, the flavonoids and the lignans, function as powerful antioxidants. If some ultraviolet energy does make it through the sunscreen layers and cause the formation of damaging free radicals in the skin, the antioxidants in Larreastat quench the free radicals before they can react with proteins or DNA and cause damage.

Regular application of Larreastat lotion under sunscreen can provide an extra level of protection from ultraviolet light to prevent cellular damage and premature aging of skin. Additionally, Larreastat capsules, taken on a daily basis, function internally to stop sun-induced free radical damage and suppress reactivation of dormant herpes viruses. For ordering information see the Source Directory starting on page 213.

Anti-aging Answers

Aging is, of course, an inevitable fact of life. But does this journey have to be a difficult one full of undesirable transitions? Or do we perhaps have more power over how we experience the passage of time than we ever realized?

In this section you will read about some anti-aging solutions that might just change your mind about the inevitability of declining eyesight, arthritis, heart disease, certain cancers, lagging libidos, and diminishing mental powers as we age. Of course these solutions don't literally stop the clock, but the tremendous effects they can have on the quality of your life might just make you feel like they do.

You will find a chapter on a powerful antioxidant that may be the answer to conquering the number one cause of blindness in the United States. You will read about a Japanese herbal combination that is thought by many to fight a number of chronic conditions including arthritis, dermatitis, and chronic fatigue—not to mention the newest research that implies that the combo might even have the ability to hinder cancer growth and slow down the aging process.

You will discover the potent anti-inflammatory antioxidant that is being credited by some experts with the ability to fight arthritis, cancer, heart disease, Alzheimers's, and indeed aging in general. You will read about a libido boosting botanical from the Amazon and we will introduce you to the powerful Ayurvedic medicine that is said to sharpen your mind and focus your memory. And finally you will learn about the once suppressed Japanese medical system that may be the powerful immunity builder that allows our Japanese counterparts to live years longer than we do.

CHAPTER 6

AstaFactor:
Powerful antioxidant, found at sea, may save you from America's leading cause of blindness

Beside the shoreline of Kona, Hawaii, an industrial-sized incubator is cultivating microscopic algae. Normally such algae would be nothing more than fish food. But this algae may yield one of the world's most potent safeguards against cancer, heart disease, and blindness.

More than 13 million Americans over the age of 40 suffer from age-related macular degeneration (ARMD). This gradual decay of the macula—a central area of the retina that provides our most acute vision—is caused by ultra-violet light, air pollution, genetics, drug use, and countless other factors that degrade eye cells. ARMD produces irreversible vision loss and ranks as the single leading cause of blindness.

Researchers at Aquasearch Inc. of Hawaii and the University of Illinois Urbana-Champaign, however, believe they've discovered a phytonutrient in the ocean that could prevent the onset of ARMD...as well as lower the risk of cancer, cardiovascular disease, and neurodegenerative diseases.

At HSI, we've been looking for something that addresses ARMD for a long time. This is the *first* promising discovery we've found, and we thought you should know about it.

Study concludes nutrient is 80 times more effective than vitamin E

Astaxanthin [as-ta-**zan**-thin] is a xanthophyll (a derivative of the pigment, carotene). It's found in certain varieties of algae and produces a pink tint in the flesh of fish that consume it (namely salmon, shrimp, crawfish, crab, lobster, and trout).

Laboratory research has demonstrated that astaxanthin has exceptional capabilities as an antioxidant (an agent that prevents the oxidation or mutation of cells) and an anti-inflammatory.[1,2] In recent animal studies at the College of Human Ecology in Seoul, Korea, astaxanthin protected the liver from toxin damage and stimulated the body's own cellular antioxidant system.[3]

Japanese researchers at the National Institute of Health and Nutrition conducted a placebo-controlled study on human subjects and found that astaxanthin inhibits the accumulation of LDL ("bad") cholesterol.[4]

Additional studies compared astaxanthin to other carotenoids and concluded that it's twice as effective as beta-carotene and nearly 80 times more effective than vitamin E at preventing oxidation within a chemical solution.[5]

Those results convinced some researchers that astaxanthin could quite capably deliver the same benefit as other antioxidants, namely lower the risk of cancer, heart disease, high cholesterol, neurodegenerative diseases, and other age-related ailments. Now, researchers also surmise that it may help you keep your sight.

ASTAXANTHIN PROTECTION GOES FARTHER THAN THE EYE CAN SEE

Even if you're not concerned about vision disorders, astaxanthin—with its ability to cross the blood-brain barrier (BBB)—may hold tremendous benefit for you.

Several confounding diseases can't be eased by supplements and drugs because those substances are stopped by the BBB. But since astaxanthin and other xanthophylls can cross the BBB to benefit the eyes, so scientists are looking into the possibility that xanthophylls may help combat diseases that involve the brain and/or the nervous system. Their research has offered some hope that astaxanthin may help relieve the symptoms or causes of Parkinson's disease, multiple sclerosis, and autoimmune disorders.

Carotenoids cross blood-brain barrier to protect eyes

To give your eyes extra protection, you may already be taking eye-specific antioxidants like lutein and zeaxanthin. Known collectively as xanthophylls, these carotenoids are found most abundantly in corn, kiwi, red seedless grapes, orange-colored peppers, spinach, celery, Brussels sprouts, scallions, broccoli, and squash.[6] And many people include these foods or xanthophyll supplements in their diets to help prevent ARMD and cataracts. (Cataracts, which sometimes appear to be caused by light-induced oxidation of eye cells, currently afflict 14 percent of Americans over the age of 40.)

What makes xanthophylls special is their ability to affect the eyes. Not all antioxidants can do that, since not all are able to cross the blood-brain barrier (BBB). The BBB is a protective mechanism designed to prevent infectious organisms and chemicals from entering the nervous system. This is an effective way to prevent illness from spreading to areas that control life itself, such as the brain. Unfortunately, it also stops beneficial substances, like many antioxidants, from protecting those same organs. Very few antioxidants can penetrate the BBB. Lutein and zeaxanthin can. And so apparently can astaxanthin.

University of Illinois researchers Mark O.M. Tso, M.D., D.Sc., and Tim-Tak Lam, Ph.D., made this key discovery in tests on rats. In a successful petition to patent astaxanthin, they state, "The administration of astaxanthin also retards the progress of degenerative eye diseases and [benefits] the vision of the individuals suffering from degenerative eye diseases, such as age-related macular degeneration."[7]

Astaxanthin levels differ by 800 percent in wild and farmed fish

One simple way to benefit from astaxanthin is to include more fish containing this xanthophyll in your diet. Salmon is the richest source. However, not all salmon have the same chance to accumulate high levels of astaxanthin. Even though aquaculture operations supplement their fish food with astaxanthin, farmed salmon have dramatically less astaxanthin than do wild salmon. Different varieties of the fish raised in different stretches of ocean also contain different levels.

For example, farm-raised Atlantic salmon fed synthetic astaxanthin contain only 0.5 mg of the antioxidant in a 4-oz serving, Free-range sockeye salmon from the North Pacific that feed on wild microalgae containing natural astaxanthin, provides about 4.5 mg in a 4-oz serving.[8] By eating the right salmon variety, you could increase your astaxanthin intake by as much as 800 percent!

Patented incubator maximizes xanthophyll's production

A potent source of astaxanthin is a microalgae called *Haemotoccus pluvialis* (H. pluvialis) that grows in the rocky coastal areas around Hawaii. Scientists at Aquasearch Inc., a local biotechnology company, have harvested samples of *H. pluvialis*, studied them, and created special cultivating techniques to maximize the microalgae's production of astaxanthin.

WATCH FOR THE WARNING SIGNS
OF MACULAR DEGENERATION AND CATARACTS

Macular degeneration is the leading cause of vision loss, with cataracts following closely behind. These eye diseases can happen any time, but they're usually associated with the natural aging process. Here are the warning signs and symptoms characteristic of these diseases:

Cataract—clouding of the eye lens

- cloudy or blurred vision
- bright lights glare, double/distorted images
- a feeling that colors aren't bright anymore
- poor night vision
- frequent changes in eyeglass or contact lens prescription

Risk factors for cataracts include smoking, diabetes, and aging.

After building high levels of the antioxidant in the microalgae, Aquasearch subjects the plant to a special churning process to break open the cells and release the astaxanthin. Next, the algae are pasteurized and dried at a low temperature, and the astaxanthin is extracted and sealed in a softgel capsule. Aquasearch markets the formula under the name AstaFactor. For ordering information see the Source Directory starting on page 213.

NIH explores potential of astaxanthin

Due to the large number of Americans who develop ARMD or cataracts, the National Institutes of Health (NIH) have also shown an interest in astaxanthin.

Barry Winkler, Ph.D., of the Eye Research Institute near Detroit, has

---

WATCH FOR THE WARNING SIGNS...*CONTINUED*

Macular degeneration—affects your central vision and can be either wet or dry (the most common variety)

- Wet—Blood vessels in the eye leak
    - straight lines appear wavy
    - rapid loss of central vision area
    - may notice a blind spot
- Dry—Deterioration of light-sensitive cells in the macula
    - blurred or blind spot in central vision area (becomes larger with time)
    - slightly blurred vision
    - need more light for reading
    - difficulty recognizing faces until they're very close

Risk factors for macular degeneration include aging, high cholesterol levels, female gender, a family history of the disease, and having fair skin and blue eyes.

---

conducted extensive research regarding the usefulness of antioxidants and carotenoids in preventing ARMD. He's currently involved in studying astaxanthin. Specifically, he is testing its ability to prevent oxidation on human retinal pigment epithelial cells that have been cultured in a lab setting. If Dr. Winkler's study shows promise, it will pave the way for a larger, prospective human clinical trial funded by the NIH to test astaxanthin's effect over a period of 10 to 15 years. We'll be sure to keep you updated in the pages of the Health Sciences Institute newsletter and through our HSI e-Alert. For information on becoming a member of HSI turn to page 223 and to sign up for the free HSI e-alert see page 225.

References

[1] Lipids, 24(7):659-61, 1989

[2] Phsiol Chem Phys Med NMR, 22(1):27-38, 1990

[3] Methods Find Exp Clin Pharmacol, 23(2):79-84, 2001

[4] J Atheroscler Throm, 7(4):216-22, 2000

[5] www.astaxanthin.org

[6] Br J Opthalmol, 82(8):907-10, 1998

[7] United States Patent No. 5,527, 533;Tso, Mark O.M. and Lam, Tim-Tak;October 27,1994

[8] J AOAC Int, 80(3):622-32,1997

CHAPTER 7

Natural Dismutase Compound:
Increase SOD levels up to 230 percent and fight arthritis, cancer, and heart disease

It's a potent anti-inflammatory and one of the most powerful antioxidants in your body. Physicians use injections of it to help cancer patients recover from radiation therapy, cardiac patients avoid further heart damage, and rheumatoid arthritis patients find relief from severe symptoms. Unfortunately, our bodies produce less of this substance as we age. (Our production actually peaks at age 10 and then falls off by about 15 percent per decade.) And researchers have regularly warned that individuals cannot substantially boost levels with supplementation.

Now, new research suggests you can dramatically augment your body's supply of this natural anti-inflammatory/antioxidant—superoxide dismutase. And enhancing your body's supply could help you combat arthritis, cancer, stroke, heart attack, Parkinson's, Alzheimer's, and aging in general. It may even provide a treatment for people struggling with Lou Gehrig's disease.

Superoxide dismutase (SOD) is an enzyme that neutralizes superoxide—a common and extremely destructive free radical. By preventing free radicals from damaging healthy cells, SOD prevents inflammation, helps prevent disease, and stops the cellular breakdown that contributes to age-related degeneration of muscles and organs.

"Old age is not old age. It is oxidative damage. It is your body failing to repair itself," says Robert Doughton, M.D., a Portland, Oregon, physician who changed his practice roughly 20 years ago to focus on alternative therapies.

Nutritionists have suggested that individuals can augment their enzyme level by eating foods rich in SOD, such as cabbage, broccoli, wheat, and barley grasses. A few SOD supplements have appeared on the market. But not much attention was given to these foods or products, since it was "proven" that SOD is destroyed by digestion. Now new research corrects that mis-interpretation.

Experience dramatic healing benefits in as little as four weeks

Researchers for SmithKline BioScience in Honolulu tested the impact of an SOD supplement on 10 individuals, aged 59 to 76. The supplement—Natural Dismutase Compound manufactured by BioMed Foods of California—is made from wheat grass biologically engineered to have high SOD content. Researchers instructed the subjects to take six capsules one hour before eating each morning for two weeks (in order to build up a loading dose), then scale back and take just three tablets each morning for the next two weeks. Blood samples drawn before and after the experiment showed that subjects' SOD levels increased 230 percent on average. (The percentage increase in each individual ranged from 32 percent to 730 percent.)[1]

According to Dr. Doughton, there are two reasons why Natural Dismutase Compound is effective orally. First, the supplement contains a huge dosage of SOD—1.6 million units per capsule. Vitamin-store SOD capsules typically contain just 400 units. Second, Natural Dismutase capsules are enterically coated, meaning they are treated to pass through the stomach unaltered and disintegrate in the intestines, thus delivering a bigger dose of SOD to the bloodstream.

BioMed recommends that individuals follow the study regimen (namely, take six capsules each morning for two weeks, then reduce the dosage to three capsules each morning). They also recommend drinking eight glasses of water per day while supplementing.

Dr. Doughton has been recommending the supplement to patients (and using it himself) since 1989. He says some rheumatoid arthritis patients who have tried Natural Dismutase have begun to experience pain relief and improved range of motion within three to four weeks of beginning supple-mentation. He notes, however, that it only works with early stage patients. "With rheumatoid arthritis, you have to supplement before you have de-formities because they are the result of unchecked oxidative damage. You can't straighten out gnarled fingers."

SOD may offer hope for "untreatable" Lou Gehrig's disease

Currently, Dr. Doughton is conducting research to determine if SOD can help people facing even more severe impairment.

The individuals most severely affected by low SOD levels are those afflicted with familial amyotrophic lateral sclerosis (ALS)—or Lou Gehrig's disease. Due to a genetic defect, they stop producing SOD altogether—a situation that accelerates damage by free radicals and results in the rapid destruction of motor neurons. In a process that has been described as "galloping old age," ALS weakens the muscles of sufferers; impedes use of their hands, arms, and legs; and makes it difficult for them to swallow or even breathe. Although a few people manage the disease long term (such as British physicist Stephen Hawkins), approximately half of all ALS sufferers die within three to five years of diagnosis.

Researchers have not yet conducted studies to determine if SOD supplements can prevent the destruction of neurons in ALS patients. Dr. Doughton, however, is developing a clinical trial to see if Natural Dismutase Compound can slow physical deterioration in people with early stage, familial ALS. If you are interested in joining the study, you can contact Dr. Doughton at (877) 635-7070.

If you're a pet owner, you know that humans aren't the only ones plagued by arthritis pain—it is also quite common in dogs and cats. The manufacturer of Natural Dismutase Compound has formulated a line of supplements specifically to ease arthritis pain in pets.

For ordering information for Natural Dismutase Compound see the Source Directory starting on page 213. As always, consult with your doctor before taking any new supplement. The supplement is not recommended for people who suffer from wheat allergies or serious morning nausea.

References
1   "Effects of whole foods on SOD deficiency" research report on www.argigenic.com

FOLLOW UP

A FOLLOW UP BRIEF FROM ROBERT DOUGHTON, MD REGARDING NATURAL DISMUTASE COMPOUND.

One of my primary interests in proposing an informal study of Natural Dismutase Compound (NDC) was to look for any possible side effects. I am happy to be able to report that out of two hundred people who took the NDC in this study, only one person, a man, complained of a rather typical itching skin rash, which did not surprise him as he was well acquainted with allergies. The side effect went away upon cessation of the supplement.

Next I was looking for the effectiveness of NDC. Unfortunately, due to a communication error regrettably a number of bottles of NDC were manufactured and distributed with half-strength tablets. However, as soon as the oversight was discovered it was corrected. While there is of course no danger in taking a half dose my concern is that many of those who took the half strength regimen, not surprisingly, would have experienced little benefit from it.

Only one person with the familial type of Lou Gherig's (ALS) disease contacted me about participating in the study and unfortunately this person was not suitable for the study as one has to be able to swallow a lot of capsules each morning (this can be very difficult for those whose swallowing muscles are weak already). As a result I am still unable to draw any final conclusions about the effectiveness of NDC on the familial form of ALS.

The study did, however, demonstrate that this product is **not**

<u>effective for the acquired form of ALS</u>. Eight persons with the acquired form of ALS received no apparent benefit to their disease with a twelve-week trial. I now feel that the *acquired* form of ALS may be akin to insulin resistant diabetes in that the problem is that they put up barriers to the dismutase (SOD) working, so it is probably not straight deficiency disease the way we believe the *familial* type is.

I am still looking for those few persons who have the familial disease, or the gene for the Amyotrophic Lateral Sclerosis disease, or the actual disease itself to try this product. This treatment is rational for such a person, affordable, preventive, and has 1/200 chance of side effects—all good reasons to give it a try.

The results of this informal study are very promising and I think they call for more in-depth study. We are still very much in business with Natural Dismutase Compound. It is remarkably effective at decreasing the aches, stiffness and pains of the muscles and joints as you age. It promotes much faster recovery from exertion. It quiets rheumatic processes and inflammation. In addition it speeds the recovery from surgical operations as far as wound healing and feeling better faster is concerned. In fact, drawing on my own observations and the results of informal study I am very comfortable stating that I believe it is a useful contribution to the antioxidant program to prevent aging. It goes without saying that to do this, it must be taken in the right dose.

For more information on NDC please see the source directory starting on page 213.

CHAPTER 8

Energy Kampo:
Stimulate your immune system, hinder cancer growth, and slow the aging process using Juzen-taiho-to

When we stumbled upon Energy Kampo, we assumed it must be a mild botanical designed to put a little extra pep in a person's day, maybe even ease the symptoms of chronic fatigue. But this product, which makes only the humble claim to help "maintain energy and well being," is actually one of Japan's most widely used herbal combinations that reportedly help the body cope with infections, disease, injury, and other stresses.

In Japan, this formulation of 10 herbal ingredients is called *Juzen-taiho-to* and is used for a wide variety of conditions. People struggling with chronic diseases (including rheumatoid arthritis, ulcerative colitis, atopic dermatitis, and chronic fatigue syndrome) take it to ease fatigue, anemia, circulatory problems, night sweats, and loss of appetite. Cancer patients take it to improve their overall condition and lessen the adverse effects of chemotherapy, radiation, and surgery.[1] It has been the subject of dozens of published studies in Asia, which have shown its potential to stimulate activity in the immune system by activating components like T-cells, lymphocytes, macrophages, spleen cells, and natural killer cells. Researchers say its immune-building properties can help people lessen the impact of lingering illness, retard the growth of cancer, and even slow the aging process.

Juzen-taiho-to proven to increase life span

Aging is caused in part by the gradual decline of T-cell activity. T-cells identify and destroy antigens (such as toxins and tumor cells) in the body, and often muster other immune responses to protect the body from disease.

One group of researchers reported that enhanced T-cell activity could even affect lifespan. Their study showed that mice fed Juzen-taiho-to lived an average of six months longer than untreated littermates.[2] On average, mice live for roughly two years; so this study showed that Juzen-taiho-to increased the average life span by 25 percent.

Treatment has potential to retard tumor growth and increase cancer survival rates

An enhanced immune system can help your body recover from any form of infection, disease, or injury. While some research and clinical practice has dealt with Juzen-taiho-to's ability to fight a range of diseases, the majority of the research has focused on the formula's potential to help cancer patients.

To our knowledge, there have not been any large-scale human trials examining the potential of Juzen-taiho-to. While researching this story, however, we found numerous published studies (all in Asian medical journals) documenting the formula's ability to retard tumor growth and metastases in laboratory animals.

At the Research Institute for Wakan-Yaku in Japan, researchers injected cancer cells into a group of mice, then gave them oral doses of Juzen-taiho-to (40 mg/day/mouse) for seven days. The treatment significantly inhibited tumor growth and prolonged survival compared to untreated mice.[3]

At the same institute, researchers set out to determine if Juzen-taiho-to could prevent colon cancer from metastasizing to the liver. They gave mice oral doses of Juzen-taiho-to for seven days prior to implanting tumors in their colons. The treatment produced a dose-dependent inhibition of cancer cells in the liver and significantly enhanced the subjects' survival rate compared to untreated mice. The treatment was not effective on mice who were already T-cell-deficient at the beginning of the experiment.[4]

However, in two separate studies, researchers documented how daily doses of Juzen-taiho-to caused old mice to develop more T cells.[5] (Curiously, one study showed the treatment did nothing to enhance the immune functions of younger mice.) The researchers reported that the treatment proved useful in correcting impaired T-cell activity in older mice and could be recommended to older humans. They concluded that "such effects of [Juzen-taiho-to] may help prevent the development of diseases…in the elderly."[6]

(continued on page 47)

THIS UNIQUE COMBINATION OF HERBS OFFERS A WEALTH OF HEALING POTENTIAL

Juzen-taiho-to is actually an ancient Chinese medicine, and was adopted by Japanese physicians during the Kamakura dynasty (1192-1333 AD). Following extensive clinical experience and pharmacological examination, the Japanese came to regard Juzen-taiho-to as a strengthening tonic for the ill and the elderly. The formulation contains the following 10 herbs, each of which has a long history and strong reputation for its healing properties.

Astragalus root (Astragali Radix)—An antiviral agent and general immune enhancer used in traditional Chinese medicine (TCM) to ease night sweats, fatigue, loss of appetite, and diarrhea. Reportedly, it helps counteract the immune-suppressing effects of cancer treatments like chemotherapy. It also helps lower blood pressure, improve circulation, and prevent heart disease.

Atractylodes Rhizome (Atractylodis Rhizoma)—A little-known TCM botanical grown mainly in Inner Mongolia, this thistle has been used to treat digestive problems, diarrhea, bloating, fatigue, as well as pain in the joints or extremities.

Chuangxiong (Cnidium Rhizome)—A TCM herb used to promote blood circulation and relieve pain.

Cinnamon bark (Cinnamomi Cortex)—Used in TCM to treat diarrhea, influenza, and parasitic worms. Cinnamon is currently taken to ease indigestion and stimulate appetite.

Dong quai (Angelicae Radix)—In TCM, dong quai is often taken as a menopause supplement (to relieve such conditions as such as hot flashes and vaginal dryness) and as a blood tonic (to regulate blood sugar and pressure, and to prevent blood clots and anemia). Studies have produced conflicting results on its efficacy and have suggested that it may work better in multi-herb formulas.

Panax ginseng (Ginseng Radix)—Traditionally, ginseng has been used to strengthen digestion, improve lung function, calm the spirit, and increase overall energy. Modern medical research has documented its potential to strengthen immunity against colds, flus and other infections; to stimulate the mind and foster a sense of well-being; and to help control diabetes and improve physical endurance.

Hoelen (Hoelen)—A botanical that reportedly acts as a diuretic and sedative, and a moderator of high blood sugar.

Licorice (Glycyrrhizae Radix) —Licorice has demonstrated abilities to act as an anti-inflammatory, cough suppressant, and anti-viral agent. It appears to increase blood flow in the stomach, possibly preventing ulcers. Recently, it has also been suggested as a possible treatment for chronic fatigue syndrome (CFS), since it mimics the action of adrenal hormones that are underactive in CFS patients. Licorice, however, contains glycyrrhiza, which can cause fluid retention, increased blood pressure, and loss of potassium.

Peony root (Paeoniae Radix)—Considered a blood tonic, it is used to correct imbalances in the blood, including poisoning, anemia, and poor circulation. It is not recommended for people with weakened livers.

Rehmannia root (Rehmanniae Radix)—An ancient Oriental botanical used to lower blood pressure and cholesterol, improve blood flow in the brain, and ease weakness. Some reports suggest it might even help avoid premature graying and baldness.

Sources: The Natural Pharmacist (www.tnp.com), "Healthy Healing," 11th edition by Linda Page, Alternatives from Nature (www.herbsrainbear.com), Herbwalk.com, Healthphone.com, and Holistic-online.com.

Not every experiment was successful, though. Studies showed that Juzen-taiho-to alone was not effective or only slightly effective in inhibiting the growth of certain varieties of melanoma, sarcoma, and fibrosarcoma (cancers of the skin, bone, and connective tissue), leukemia and Lewis lung carcinoma.

Formula increases power, lessens side effects of chemotherapy

While no one has suggested this 10-herb formula can replace radiation, chemotherapy, or surgery, preliminary research suggests Juzen-taiho-to can increase the power of conventional cancer treatment and lessen some of its worst side effects.

At Toyama Medical and Pharmaceutical University in Japan, researchers tested the ability of Juzen-taiho-to and the cancer drug interferon alpha (IFN-alpha) to prevent renal (kidney cell) cancer from metastasizing to the lungs of laboratory mice. They found that the combination of both treatments offered much greater results for inhibiting metastasis than either treatment had alone. Furthermore, the combined treatment did not induce any weight loss—one of the negative side effects associated with IFN-alpha therapy."[7]

Other studies reported that the combination of Juzen-taiho-to and conventional cancer drugs inhibited the growth of sarcoma, melanoma, fibrosarcoma, bladder cancer, colon cancer, leukemia, and abdominal tumors more effectively than either the formula or the drug could individually."[8,9]

The combination can also ameliorate the side effects of treatment. In several studies, Japanese researchers found that mice treated orally with Juzen-taiho-to for one to two weeks before receiving conventional cancer drug treatment suffered fewer side effects. Liver and kidney toxicity was significantly reduced, and the animals didn't lose as many blood cells and platelets or as much body weight as untreated mice. Overall, their immune systems remained stronger and their survival times were longer.

Juzen-taiho-to is sold in the United States under the label Energy Kampo. For ordering information see the Source Directory starting on page 213.

References

[1] Bio Pharm Bull, 23(6): 677-88, 2000

[2] J Invest Dermatol, 117(3):694-701, 2002

[3] Jpn J Cacner Res, 87(10): 1,039-44, 1996

[4] Jpn J Cacner Res, 89(2): 206-13, 1998

[5] Mech Ageing Dev, 122(3): 341-52, 2001

[6] Am J Chin Med, 27(2): 191-203, 1999

[7] Anticancer Res, 20(5A): 2,931-7, 2000

[8] Bio Pharm Bull, 23(6): 677-88, 2000

[9] Gan To Kagaku Ryoho, 16(4 Pt 2-2): 1,500-5, 1989

CHAPTER 9

Clavo Huasca:

By special request: Something to spice up the ladies' nights

...by Health Sciences Institute panelist Leslie Taylor

It was probably more fun than any "guinea pig" in any medical experiment ever had before.

As part of my work with Raintree Nutrition, I organized an informal clinical trial last year. I was about to introduce a new product—a natural libido enhancer for women. Although I had learned enough about its medical track record to be convinced of its effectiveness, I wanted to test it on some women. So I enlisted the help of a psychotherapist in Austin, Texas. She was running several support groups (dealing with women and money, women and relationships, those kinds of issues) so she had access to lots of willing participants and the means to track the results of a test. She recruited a total of 75 women ranging in age from early 30s to early 60s, distributed the product to them, and then got them to report on their reactions to it at the end of each weekly therapy session.

The stories sounded like something out of a romance novel. According to their first-hand reports, many of the women were waking up in the middle of the night with erotic dreams. Some even had spontaneous orgasms. And they said it made them more aggressive sexually, on a mental level. They just thought about sex more often, were more assertive in making the first move, and ultimately enjoyed the experience more.

Like all of the products from Raintree, the libido enhancer is a botanical from the Amazon rain forest that has long been used by traditional healers there. But to find this little gem, I had to overcome an unexpected challenge.

Teaching feminism to Indian shamans

I work with a lot of Indian shamans to learn about medicinal plants found in the rainforest and the natural plant remedies traditionally made from them. One of the first products that I launched was a sexual stimulant for men. The shamans, herbalists, and many other people I encountered in South America were entirely comfortable talking about sexual function and performance where men were concerned. But for the longest time, I couldn't get the shamans to trust me enough to tell me what they used as a sexual stimulant for women. I didn't realize it at first, but I had run into a cultural roadblock. Many communities in the Amazon are still traditional patriarchal societies. Women are often regarded as vessels who wouldn't even consider saying no to their husbands. In that kind of society, a woman's satisfaction with her own sex life isn't even remotely important.

But I pursued the topic further. I explained the cultural difference to the shamans. I told them that in Western societies, men actually like women who have strong libidos. Then finally, the shamans opened up and began sharing their knowledge. They told me about several plants that enhanced female libido and sexual performance. But over and over, their discussion kept swinging back to one particular plant.

Clavo huasca is a large, woody vine, indigenous to the Amazon rain forest, that can grow up to 80 meters in length. Its bark which is used in therapeutic preparations, has a strong clove-like aroma. Consequently, it is commonly known as the Clove Vine.

In Peruvian herbal medicine, *Clavo huasca* is widely regarded as an aphrodisiac for both men and women. It's a main ingredient in two old and still popular formulas for impotency and frigidity that are sold in herbal markets around Peru—*Siete raices* (Seven Roots) and *Rompe Calzon* (Bust your Britches).

Feel "friskier" in as little as one week

My *Clavo huasca* product is simply a highly concentrated extract of the vine (1 milliliter of extract is equivalent to 500 mg of *Clavo huasca* vine) blended with 40 percent alcohol to stabilize and preserve the active ingredients. (And no, the preparation does not contain enough alcohol to induce any amorous thoughts—not unless you're capable of becoming inebriated on a single dropperful of alcohol.)

As yet, there are no published clinical trials on the medicinal actions of *Clavo huasca*. And frankly, I can't tell you just how it works, since I'm not entirely sure myself. I just know from numerous reports from women both in South America and the United States that it does indeed seem to work.

By all accounts, it seems to provide sexual stimulation mentally rather than doing anything physiological to improve sexual function. But to be honest with you, I think women's libido is more deeply rooted in their minds and in their psyches than men's anyway. Roughly 85 percent of the women I know who have tried *Clavo huasca*, have had a positive experience with it. (By contrast, only 20 percent of men have benefited from it. Directly, that is.)

On average, women begin to feel effects from it within a week or two of beginning the supplement. After it begins working, some women find that continued daily doses generate too much libido (though I'd be willing to bet most of their husbands would say there's no such thing), and have reported that one dose every two to three days is better for them.

It doesn't work for everybody. It will not help women who need a uterine relaxant or something to ease vaginal dryness. Likewise, it is not effective for post-menopausal or post-pregnancy women who are having libido problems due to hormonal imbalances. To date, however, there have been no reports of it generating adverse side effects and I have found no reason to believe it is contraindicated for individuals with any particular medical conditions. Of course, certain individuals shouldn't consume alcohol due to health conditions or medications. If you are in that situation, consult with your doctor before trying *Clavo huasca* to determine if you can safely ingest 12 drops of alcohol daily (the amount found in a full dose). Or if you'd just rather avoid consuming alcohol, add your daily dose to two to three ounces of just-boiling water, then let the mixture cool before consuming it. The heat will cause most of the alcohol to evaporate.

So if the mood strikes you, go ahead and try it. There's no reason the "guinea pigs" should have all the fun!

See the Source Directory starting on page 213 for information on ordering clavo huasca.

FOLLOW UP

CAN CLAVO HUASCA JUMPSTART A STALLED SEX LIFE? THE RESULTS ARE IN...

Recently, we told our HSI members and e-Alert readers about an exciting new product from Raintree Nutrition called *clavo huasca* (see page 223 for HSI membership information). According to Indian shamans, it can help women "spice up" their sex lives. Leslie Taylor, one of our HSI panelists and the founder and president of Raintree Nutrition, Inc., told us about this new find from the Amazon, and shared the results of an informal *clavo* trial she conducted with 75 women. Her findings were very positive, so we were excited to bring this information to our female members, who have been asking for something like this for a long, long time.

In fact, we decided to form our own informal test group, and through an e-Alert (see page 225 for information on signing up for the free HSI e-Alert service), we invited women over the age of 50 to contact us if they wanted to participate. Raintree Nutrition, Inc., provided free one-month supplies of *clavo huasca* to all participants, and we asked them to keep a journal and submit weekly reports of the effects.

The results are in—and, though the benefits aren't as widespread as we had hoped, they're not at all disappointing. The 38 women who participated in the study from start to finish split right down the middle—19 experienced no changes, and 19 reported benefits. Of these, six said the benefits were slight, while 13 felt that the herb improved their sexual relations.

We weren't entirely surprised because Ms. Taylor told us that *clavo huasca* doesn't work for everybody. In fact, in the August issue she specifically noted that *clavo* would not help women who need a uterine relaxant, or women who suffer with vaginal dryness or hormone imbalances. While we tried to control for those situations, some of those conditions might explain the results of our trial.

"THE BEST SEX I'VE HAD IN AGES..."

But the 13 women who did see major benefits submitted some dramatic reports—not the standard type of reports we read here at HSI, in case you're wondering. Susan T. wrote, "I think I am more receptive toward sex and I do think about it more often...I am more inclined to daydream about sex, and yes, I have started to think about romantic situations." Alice H. wrote, "WOW, I had a very erotic dream that was vivid and color-ful. The next day I had the best sex I have had in ages. Outstanding, great, wonderful." Joan M. wrote, "I can't believe I am almost 67 years old with a 72-year-old lover and we are behaving like sex-crazed kids. It is fun...I am enjoying it A LOT...My thoughts about this product are very positive. More intense sex. Increased desire for sex. Orgasms that are very strong and last longer."

Some of the participants also reported other positive benefits of *clavo*—even when they didn't feel a change in their libido. Women said they slept better, had a better attitude, and had more energy. And none of the women reported any side effects from taking clavo.

But many also said that they didn't enjoy the taste of *clavo*, which is delivered in a liquid extract. We asked Ms. Taylor about that, and she recommended adding the liquid drops to juice, particularly cranberry juice, to mask the taste.

The results of the trial weren't quite what we had hoped for. But *clavo* clearly made a difference for some women. If you decide to try *clavo*, we'd love to hear about your results (see the Source Directory starting on page 213 for ordering information). In the meantime, we'll continue to search for other natural libido boosters, and bring you the information as soon as we find it.

CHAPTER 10

Liver Kampo:
Japanese medical system, once forced underground, may hold the secret to a longer, healthier life

Japanese health and longevity rates have confounded envious onlookers for years. On average, Japanese men live four years longer than American men; Japanese women live five years longer than their American counterparts.[1] Now, you can benefit from one of the secrets of their success.

Kampo, also known as Japanese herbal medicine, is an ancient system of healing that has been professionalized, subjected to Western standards of pharmaceutical research, and integrated into modern Japanese medicine. Today, almost half of Japan's medical schools instruct students in Kampo and 78 percent of Japanese physicians regularly prescribe Kampo preparations for their patients.[2] And research is mounting that Kampo's whole-herb, pharmaceutical-grade supplements are capable of warding off colds, easing upset stomachs, neutralizing the effects of menopause, treating liver disease, and even inhibiting the growth of cancers.

Public demand brings underground medicine back to mainstream hospitals

Kampo is derived from traditional Chinese medicine (TCM), although it's not nearly as well known in the Western world.

First introduced in Japan between the sixth and eighth centuries, traditional Chinese medicine was widely accepted by Japanese physicians—who adapted the system and modified many of its formulas to create Kampo medicine.

Kampo constituted the official medical system of Japan until the start of the Meiji era (1866-1912), when Emperor Mutsuhito came to power and embraced Western medical practices. While Kampo was not completely replaced by "modern" medicine, it was eventually forced to an "underground" status after Japan instituted a physician-licensing practice that certified doctors only if they were educated in Western-style medicine.

Due largely to public demand, Kampo was integrated back into the medical mainstream in the 1960s. Japanese physicians began to combine the ancient medical wisdom with the rigors of modern medical research. The Japanese government enacted legislation requiring manufacturers of Kampo formulas to meet the same quality standards as pharmaceutical companies. It also extended the national medical insurance to cover Kampo formulas. By 1990, Japanese consumers were buying 1.5 billion bottles of Kampo products annually.

The secret to Kampo's success?
Mixing the herbs, *then* making the extract

The botanical ingredients used in Kampo's 210 formulas are often the same ingredients found in TCM formulations. However, Kampo preparations usually contain <u>lower</u> concentrations of active constituents than their TCM counterparts.[3] This does not mean Kampo medicines are inferior or ineffective. In fact, the opposite may be true.

Both Kampo and TCM supplements start with the whole herb. However, the processing of that herb is what separates these two traditional medicines. TCM supplements use individual herbs and make extracts of each before combining them. Kampo, on the other hand, combines whole herbs and then makes an extract of the compounded formula. This unique method of formulation allows Kampo medicine to use <u>reduced dosages without sacrificing effectiveness</u>.

With 210 formulations, Kampo medicine is too expansive a topic to cover in one newsletter. While we expect to focus on other formulas in future issues of the HSI Members Alert and the HSI e-Alerts (see pages 223 and 225 for information on becoming a member of the Health Sciences Institute and for signing up for free HSI e-Alerts), we'll begin by investigating one of the most widely used—Liver Kampo. Liver Kampo is a compound of seven medicinal plants reported to build immunity, foster liver health, treat cirrhosis and hepatitis, and inhibit the growth of several kinds of cancer.

Do *you* have a healthy liver?

Liver function can be compromised by a number of things—pollution, pharmaceuticals, pesticides, steroids, poor diet, insufficient rest, stress, obesity, smoking, and illness, to name a few. Since the liver is one of the most important organs when it comes to fighting illness, liver problems can have serious consequences. And, with a list of threats to your liver like that, developing an unhealthy one is more common than you may think.

Living with a weakened liver is akin to putting out the "welcome mat" for viruses, bacteria, and other disease-causing microbes, which can lead to life-threatening illnesses. Ordinarily, your liver filters these microorganisms from your bloodstream. (Blood, containing bacteria, enters the liver and comes in contact with Kupffer cells. In less than 0.01 seconds, the bacteria passes through the cell wall and lodges there until it is digested. The blood exits the liver sterile.[4]) But if it's overworked or not functioning optimally, it can't do its job properly and some organisms pass through, resulting in illness.

If you catch a lot of colds or come down with whatever variety of flu is making the rounds each winter, it may be caused by a weakened liver and consequently a weakened immune system.

Sho-saiko-to, also known as SST or Liver Kampo, addresses the core of many types of illnesses—inadequate or low immunity. While Western medicine often treats the symptoms of a disease, Liver Kampo addresses the body's entire response to illness and bolsters it so illness cannot get a foothold.

Halt or slow the progression of hepatitis C

Recent statistics show that more than 1.5 million Japanese patients with chronic liver disease have been treated with Liver Kampo. While a number of mechanisms may be responsible for its beneficial effects, Japanese scientists at Mie University School of Medicine believe an increase in interleukin-12 (IL-12) may be one of the keys to its health benefits. (Interleukin is a substance that stimulates the disease-fighting abilities of the immune system.)

To test this theory, researchers measured the interleukin-12 levels of 11 patients with hepatitis-C virus (HCV) and compared them with the inter-leukin levels in 12 healthy subjects. Those suffering from HCV showed "significantly lower" levels than the healthy patients. When the researchers added Liver Kampo to the laboratory sample for the hepatitis patients, IL-12 production levels "increased approximately three fold" and became "almost the same as those from healthy subjects."[5]

Another study indicates that hepatitis C patients may be able to slow down the progress of their disease by supplementing with Liver Kampo and consequently regulating their interleukin production. Scientists from the Department of Laboratory Medicine at Mie University found that blood samples from HCV sufferers had high levels of IL-4 and IL-5 and low levels

---

THE SECRET TO HUNDREDS OF YEARS OF HEALING

Liver Kampo's formula has stayed the same for hundreds of years, because it has repeatedly proven successful. While the ingredients work synergistically, they are also quite potent individually. The seven active ingredients and their actions include the following:

- **Bupleurum root:** reduces adhesion of tumor cells,[7] activates natural defenses against tumor cells,[8] and reduces Parkinson's tremor[9]

- **Pinellia tuber:** increases interferon activity[10]

- **Ginger:** inhibits the spread of cancer cells[11]

- **Scutellaria root:** scavenges free radicals,[12] relaxes blood vessels, reduces blood pressure,[13] and exhibits antitumor activity[14]

- **Jujube:** increases natural killer cell activity[15] and is antiasthmatic[16]

- **Ginseng:** inhibits cancer cell growth by suppressing their DNA[17] and increases natural immune factors[18]

- **Licorice:** generates interferon activity,[19] protects the gastric system,[20] is chemopreventive,[21] reduces Parkinson's tremor,[22] and has antiviral activity[23]

of IL-10 as compared with normal levels found in non-HCV patients. However, the addition of Liver Kampo resulted in an increase in IL-10 and a 25 percent to 33 percent decrease in IL-4 and IL-5 levels. The researchers concluded that Liver Kampo "may be useful in the prevention of [HCV] progression."[6]

Kampo combination forces tumor-causing cells to die, preventing cancer growth

In an article that reviewed the benefits of botanicals, researchers from the Department of Pharmacology and Therapeutics at Seth GS Medical College in India cite the unique ability of plants to increase the rate of death of cancerous cells. While they wrote in general terms about herbal therapies and drug extracts of many plants, they specifically cited Liver Kampo as a formulation that can force tumor-causing cells to die.[24] This is an important prelude to preventing cancer growth, since one of the disease's growth mechanisms is to mutate cells so they exceed their normal life span.

The researchers based their comments on several studies, including one conducted at the Nagoya University School of Medicine in Japan. Researchers there determined that the combination of herbs in Liver Kampo is stronger than any one of the individual components alone in preventing metastatic activity and thereby suppressing tumor development.[25]

At the School of Medicine at Yamaguchi University in Japan, researchers found that Liver Kampo could prevent preneoplastic lesions in the livers of mature male rats by inhibiting the activation of stellate cells.[26] Researchers concluded that inhibiting these cells might lead to a "reduction in the development of preneoplastic lesions"(abnormal tissue growths that could become cancerous). This mechanism is different than most mainstream cancer fighters, because it appears to stop the carcinogenic process in an extremely early stage before it can make any substantial headway.

Other research indicated that Liver Kampo seems able to inhibit the progression of kidney cancer. Researchers at the School of Medicine at Keio University in Tokyo tested the herbal combination on mice suffering from renal cell carcinoma. They administered both Liver Kampo and interleukin-2 to the mice for 30 days (the mice received 2.5 grams of Liver Kampo per kilogram of body weight) and found that the combination "inhibited growth of the tumor and prolonged survival significantly when compared with untreated mice."[27]

Eliminate chronic ailments and allergies

Besides fighting cancer, you can derive many other health benefits by boosting your liver function. Traditionally, Liver Kampo has been recommended for a number of chronic health problems, including gastroenteritis, hepatitis, and tonsillitis. It has been traditionally prescribed for orthostatic hypotension (low blood pressure that occurs when you stand after sitting or lying down). It has also been used to treat bronchial asthma.[28]

Because asthma attacks can be induced by allergies, reducing the body's reaction to allergens is a big step in eliminating this disorder. Doctors at Izumiotsu Municipal Hospital in Osaka, Japan conducted a test on cells extracted from laboratory rats. They tried to stimulate an allergic reaction (specifically, a release of histamine) by exposing the cells to an antigen. Three hours after the herbal complex was administered, no histamine was released—confirming that Liver Kampo "has an active anti-allergic effect."[29]

Cirrhosis patients live longer, avoid liver cancer

One of the largest human studies of Liver Kampo was conducted by the Osaka City University Medical School in Japan. It involved 260 patients with liver cirrhosis and hepatitis B. The subjects were assigned to either a control group that received only conventional treatment or a group that received Liver Kampo supplements (7.5 grams each) in tandem with conventional treatment. The groups were matched for age, sex, severity of illness, and the presence of hepatitis B antigens. The subjects received treatment and were followed for five years to determine if there were any long-term effects or benefits from receiving Kampo medicine. The researchers found that the "survival curve for five years of the trial group was higher than that of the control group." Because cirrhosis of the liver has a very high probability of developing into liver cancer, it is important to stop this life-threatening process. The scientists concluded that Liver Kampo "helped prevent the development of [liver cancer] in patients with cirrhosis."[30]

Other research suggests this Kampo formula may also help patients recover from liver surgery.[31]

Good digestion essential to benefiting from Liver Kampo

There is one trick to realizing the benefit of Liver Kampo: Your body must be able to absorb the formula's nutrients quickly and transfer those nutrients into your bloodstream before your digestive system expels them. One way to ensure fast absorption is to maintain healthy bowel flora.[32] Recent research from New Zealand shows that a decline in beneficial bacteria occurs with normal aging. The research has also determined that supplementing with a probiotic containing bifidobacteria can increase nutrient absorption and help restore some lost immune function.[33] In order to get the most out of supplementing with Liver Kampo, you might want to consider taking a supplement that contains live bifidobacteria.

Liver Kampo is imported by Honso USA, Inc. a division of Honso Pharmaceutical Co. Ltd. in Japan, and can be purchased through BenSalem Naturals in Pennsylvania. For ordering information see the Source Directory starting on page 213.

Diabetes and pneumonia patients need to exercise caution

Because Liver Kampo affects your entire body, and not just isolated symptoms, it may also affect some medications you are taking. Japanese

(continued on page 62)

AN UNEXPECTED WAY TO PREVENT ULCERS

One interesting health benefit of Liver Kampo has nothing to do with immune protection. Scientists found that the herbal complex has the ability to protect the mucous tissue and muscle lining the digestive tract. While it's not entirely clear what mechanism generates this protection, an animal study conducted by the Central Research Laboratories at Tsumura & Co., in Ibaraki, Japan, shows that it can protect against ulcers that may be caused by drugs or stress.[34]

scientists with the Department of Pharmacy at Shimane Medical University Hospital in Izumo assayed the botanical ingredients of Liver Kampo and found that one of its constituents (licorice) adversely affects tolbutamide, a medication used for the treatment of diabetes.[35] If you are diabetic or take any type of diabetes medication, consult your health care practitioner before using Liver Kampo or any other preparation containing licorice (glycyrrhizae radix) or one of its active constituents (glycyrrhizin).

If you have a tendency to get pneumonia or chest colds or are suffering from any type of lung disorder, consult your physician before using Liver Kampo. While this formula has been safely used for hundreds of years by millions of people, medical reports from the past 10 years show pneumonia,[36] pneumonitis,[37] and pulmonary edema[38] have occasionally developed after Liver Kampo supplementation. Scientists are unsure why Liver Kampo may cause or aggravate these illnesses, but their occurrences are extremely rare.

References

[1] World Health Organization, World Health Statistics Annual, 1997-99

[2] Academic Medicine, 75(1):1-2, 2000

[3] J Ethnopharmacology, 73(1-2):1-13, 2000

[4] Guyton & Hall Textbook of Medical Physiology, 9th edition, page 885

[5] Dev Immunol, 7(1):17-22, 1999

[6] Hepatology, 25(6):1390-7, 1997

[7] Planta Med, 64(3):220-4, 1998

[8] Immunopharmacology, 30(1):79-87, 1995

[9] Psychiatry Clin Neurosci, 54(5):579-82, 2000

[10] Int J Immunopharmacol, 15(2):237-43, 1993

[11] Anticancer Res, 17(2A):873-8, 1997

[12] Biol Pharm Bull, 24(10):1202-5, 2001

[13] Biol Pharm Bull, 24(10):1137-41, 2001

[14] Urology, 55(6):951-5, 2000

[15] Biol Pharm Bull, 19(7):936-9, 1996

[16] Exp Lung Res, 22(3):255-66, 1996

[17] Jpn J Cancer Res, 92(11):1184-9, 2001

[18] Antibiot Khimioter, 46(7):19-22, 2001

[19] Int J Immunopharmacol, 15(2):237-43, 1993

[20] Comp Biochem Physiol C. Pharmacol Toxicol Endocrinol, 113(1):17-21, 1996

[21] Mutat Res, 480-1:201-7, 2000

[22] Psychiatry Clin Neurosci, 54(5):579-82, 2000

[23] Am J Chin Med, 27(1):53-62, 1999

[24] Cell Mol Biol (Niosy-le-grand), 46(1):199-214, 2000

References...*continued*

[25] J Invest Dermatol, 111(4):640-4, 1998

[26] J Hepatol, 28(2):298-306, 1998

[27] Keio J Med, 46(3):132-7, 1997

[28] J Ethnopharmacol, 73(1-2):1-13, 2000

[29] Eur Arch Otorhinolaryngol, 255(7):359-64, 1998

[30] Cancer, 76(5):743-9, 1995

[31] J Pharm Pharmacol, 52(1):111-8, 2000

[32] Bio Pharm Bull, 21(12):1251-7, 1998

[33] http://www.lef.org/whatshot/#bphr

[34] Bio Pharm Bull, 20(11):1155-9, 1997

[35] Bio Pharm Bull, 24(4):409-13, 2001

[36] Nihon Kyobu Shikkan Gakkai Zasshi, 35(12):1372-7, 1997

[37] Nihon Kyobu Shikkan Gakkai Zasshi, 37(5):396-400, 1999

[38] Nihon Kyobu Shikkan Gakkai Zasshi, 36(9):776-80, 1998

MindCare:
Focus your mind, sharpen your memory with Ayurvedic medicine

Year after year, the car keys seem to go missing more often. Names of distant relatives and household gadgets don't jump to mind the instant you need them. Memories of family events grow hazy. Tasks like balancing the checkbook or preparing a holiday meal become more challenging and more prone to errors. And one day you start wondering if you're edging down that path toward dementia.

Practitioners of Ayurvedic (traditional Indian) medicine, however, have identified several herbs capable of preserving memory and mental acuity and even reversing some age-related cognitive deficits. Practitioners say these herbs, which have been used for centuries, can offset the prime causes of memory loss, namely disease, nerve cell decay, nutritional deficiencies, and stress.

It's a nasty biological fact that our capacity to maintain a sharp memory diminishes as we age. On average, individuals lose nerve cells at a rate of 1 percent a year after age 25. Consequently by age 70, we've lost more than one-third of the cells critical to memory functions. Memory loss can be exacerbated by other factors: stress, depression, disease (including diabetes and hypothyroidism), nutritional deficiencies (especially of vitamins B_1 and B_{12}), and certain prescription medications. Trauma, strokes, and heart attacks can reduce oxygen flow to the brain, killing cells and causing memory loss. Sadly, Alzheimer's disease also causes extreme memory loss in one in 10 Americans over the age of 65.

Several Ayurvedic herbs, however, support the brain directly. Bacopa, for example, affects higher-order cognitive processes by rejuvenating nerves and brain cells.[1] Gotu kola helps maintain microvessels in the brain, improving memory and attention span.[2] Mucuna is a natural source of levodopa that optimizes performance of the nervous system, including the brain.[3]

Others bolster cognitive function by strengthening the nervous system. Ashwaganda (or Indian ginseng) fights stress,[4] improves memory,[5] and helps rejuvenate people suffering from general debility, exhaustion, or stress-induced fatigue. Salep orchid is a nerve stimulant. And Morning Glory is an anti-aging remedy that improves memory and intellect by easing nervous debility.

A few herbs also help individuals suffering from memory loss or concentration problems brought on by stress. Muskroot, for example, is a nerve tonic known for its calming effect on the mind.[6]

Now studies indicate that certain Ayurvedic herbs might even offer positive results for severe conditions like Alzheimer's disease and amnesia.

THE RIGHT DIET MAY PRESERVE YOUR MEMORY

There are a number of things you can do to regain some lost mental function and improve your concentration. Daily exercise is an excellent way to increase circulation, which helps relieve mind-numbing stress and increase oxygen flow to the brain. Herbs like ginseng and Ginkgo biloba have been used for centuries in many cultures and appear to increase the amount of oxygen-rich blood to the brain. Supplements like phosphatidylserine and NADH are more recent discoveries that have been found to keep the brain sharp and functioning at its peak. Finally, a diet that includes ample raw fruit and vegetables (the best sources of antioxidants), sufficient protein (which helps maintain nerve cells and healthy blood sugar levels), and cold-water fish (which contain Omega-3 fatty acids and reduce the risk of strokes, blood clots, and heart attacks) protect against many diseases that impair cognitive function. Adding 500-1,000 mg of l-carnitine greatly helps transport these essential fatty acids into cells.

Laboratory tests reveal potential to treat amnesia and Alzheimer's

Scientists at the National Institute of Mental Health and Neuroscience in Bangalore, India, investigated the ability of one formula to treat amnesia. MindCare, a formulation by Himalaya USA, contains all of the herbs mentioned above as well as Indian valerian (a calming agent) and two herbs that protect against memory-damaging diseases: Guduchi (a tonic that bolsters natural immunity[7]) and Triphala (a combination of three Ayurvedic herbs high in vitamins B and C, which can be depleted by stress). The scientists administered MindCare to laboratory rats suffering from amnesia induced by electroshock therapy. In the medical journal Probe, the researchers reported that MindCare "enhances cognition against...amnesia."[8]

Researchers at the Institute of Medical Sciences at Banaras Hindu University in India found that lab rats suffering from cognitive decline due to Alzheimer's disease also responded positively to MindCare supplementation. After two weeks of supplementation, the rats experienced a reversal of cognitive deficits.[9] The researchers discovered heightened concentrations of acetylcholine in the rats' brains—a condition that improves cognitive processes and memory.

Ease the anxiety that can cloud memories and impair concentration

In other studies, MindCare has demonstrated abilities to ease the stress and anxiety that can exacerbate memory and concentration problems. At the Baranas Hindu University in Varanasi, India, researchers gave rats MindCare for seven days. Afterward, the rats received a drug that increases tribulin—a marker in the brain that indicates the subject is suffering from anxiety. The researchers found that pretreatment with MindCare attenuated the effects of the anxiety-causing drug.[10]

Doctors at Varanasi's Institute of Medical Sciences in India conducted a memory and anxiety test on 20 individuals age 15 to 65. In their study, which was published in the medical journal *Probe*, test subjects received either two placebos or two MindCare tablets twice a day for 12 weeks. The

(continued on page 69)

RESEARCHERS INVESTIGATE POSSIBLE TREATMENT FOR ADD

Research suggests that MindCare might also benefit children and young adults suffering from attention deficit disorder (ADD) or simple concentration problems.

In one study, 50 students at the Banaras Hindu University took either two placebos or two MindCare tablets three times a day for three months to determine if the formula could help them stay focused on their studies. Researchers tested the students' concentration at both the beginning and the end of the study. Both groups posted improved scores on the post-study tests. However, the students treated with MindCare registered an improvement that was three times greater than the improvement among those taking placebos.[12]

In 1990, doctors attending the First National Conference of the Indian Psychiatric Society's Child and Adolescent Mental Health Sub-speciality reported on another MindCare study. Sixty children who participated in a double-blind, placebo-controlled study received either a placebo or MindCare for 12 weeks. The students were tested initially, again after six weeks, and finally after 12 weeks. Scientists noted that most of the improvements for the MindCare group were noticeable within the first six weeks of treatment and then progressed further during the second half of the study. They concluded that the students receiving MindCare "responded significantly well" and "did better on the parameters of attention, hyperactivity, impulsivity, tractability, academics, language development, and fine motor functioning" than students receiving placebos. Those receiving placebos showed some improvement after the first six weeks of the study, but did not demonstrate any further improvement in behavior during the second six weeks.[13]

Himalaya USA has developed a special formula for children called MindCare Jr. It contains the same ingredients as MindCare but is formulated specifically for children and packaged in smaller tablets. For ordering information see the Source Directory starting on page 213.

subjects then took a word test to determine the supplement's effect on short-term memory. The individuals taking MindCare showed a 10-point improvement over pre-treatment memory tests. The placebo group improved by approximately two points. The MindCare group registered a similar improvement in anxiety testing. Researchers found "there was a statistically significant decrease" in anxiety after taking MindCare, but the group taking placebos showed no improvement in their anxiety levels.[11]

MindCare is available through Himalaya USA. For ordering information see the Source Directory starting on page 213.

References
1 Psychopharmacology (Berl), 156(4):481-4, 2001
2 Angiology, 52 Suppl 2:S9-13, 2001
3 J Altern Complement Med, 1(3):249-55, 1995
4 Phytother Res, 15(6):544-8, 2001
5 Phytother Res, 15(6):524-8, 2001
6 Arzneimittelforschung, 28(1):7-13, 1978
7 J Ethnopharmacology, 54(2-3):119-24, 1996
8 Probe, 37(3):179-81, 1998
9 Fitoterapia, 66(3):216-22, 1995
10 Indian Journal of Experimental Biology, 32(1):37-43, 1994
11 Mentat (MindCare) Product Monograph, pages 131-2
12 Mentat (MindCare) Product Monograph, pages 129-30
13 Probe, 30(3):227-32, 1991

Breathing Free

Experts tell us that the average person reaches his peak lung capacity in his mid twenties at which point he then starts to gradually lose that capacity. According to one breathing development expert, while 99 percent of our energy <u>should be</u> coming from breathing, most of us only access 10% to 20 % of our breathing capacity.

When we are unable to properly oxygenate our bodies our health inevitably suffers as a result. Almost every conceivable disease or illness can be improved upon, or be caused to worsen, depending on our ability to breathe well. Breathing is at the very core of our health and well being.

In this section you will be introduced to a couple of solutions to the breathing difficulties that you or a loved one may be experiencing. You will read about the incredible research behind a targeted breathing method that has been shown in many cases to treat asthma symptoms even <u>better</u> than drugs or supplements. These techniques, simple enough to be taught to a child, can help improve your blood oxygenation levels which can have long-lasting positive effects even for those not currently suffering from an asthmatic condition.

You will also discover how a specific enzyme, found in nature, might have the ability to ease all sorts of inflammations particularly those related to respiratory illnesses including allergic reactions and bronchitis. The anti-inflammatory actions of this substance may have far reaching benefits for a variety of other medical conditions as well.

CHAPTER 12

Buteyko Home Education Kit:
Targeted breathing method shown to treat asthma better than drugs or supplements

While mainstream treatments try to "control" asthma by throwing bronchodilators and steroids at the symptoms, an alternative therapy developed by a Russian doctor has actually <u>eliminated the cause of asthma in over 90 percent of patients</u>. For the 17 million Americans suffering with asthma, this may finally provide them with true relief.

Nine out of 10 of us breathe <u>incorrectly</u>—and we may be sick because of it

In the 1940s, Professor Konstantin Pavlovich Buteyko (byew-TAY-ko) of the then-Soviet Union observed that only 10 percent of all people breathe correctly and that asthma is just one of many health problems caused by improper breathing. Through his observation of hospitalized asthma patients, Dr. Buteyko concluded that the majority of asthma attacks are triggered by patients breathing too quickly.

Hyperventilation, or overbreathing, is the process of taking several breaths in the same period of time that a normal person would take one breath. Dr. Buteyko discovered that asthma sufferers take three to four breaths when they should be taking only one. And this process can start a cascade of events that eventually leads to asthma and other health problems.

Hyperventilation decreases the oxygen sent to your bloodstream

The more breaths you take in a short period of time, the less oxygen is available to your bloodstream. Your lungs require a certain amount of time to process the air you inhale. Hyperventilation short-circuits this mechanism and deprives your body of the time it needs to process each breath. And for each extra breath you take, the amount of available oxygen drops that much more. It's a classic case of diminishing returns when the next breath follows too closely on the heels of the previous one.

In addition to reducing oxygen in the blood, hyperventilation also decreases your levels of carbon dioxide (CO_2) and may cause a deficiency of the gas. A low level of CO_2 drops your body's pH level and creates an alkaline environment, which encourages viral growth and allergies. Recurring infections and multiple allergies are common in asthma victims and often complicate treatment efforts.

CO_2 also plays an important role in dilating smooth muscles, including those in your lungs. This is believed to be one of the mechanisms that initiates bronchial spasms in asthma sufferers.

Even though too little CO_2 compromises blood-oxygen levels, simply supplying CO_2 to asthma sufferers doesn't prevent or stop asthmatic attacks.[1] What Dr. Buteyko found was that you *can* increase levels of oxygen and CO_2 and effectively prevent and stop asthma attacks by learning controlled breathing techniques.

Traditional asthma treatment *increases* drug use

The claims made by Dr. Buteyko were especially interesting to officials of the Australian Association of Asthma Foundations, since surveys show that nine percent of Australian adults have asthma and up to 20 percent of Australian children suffer from it. As a result, researchers conducted a prospective, placebo-controlled, randomized, blind study at Brisbane's Mater Hospital to determine if the Buteyko method could decrease or shorten asthma attacks better than conventional methods.

Thirty-nine severe asthmatics ages 12 to 70 were placed into either a treatment group or a placebo group and received 90 minutes of training a day for seven days. While the treatment group was taught the Buteyko method of breathing, the control group received traditional asthma treatment—which the hospital doctors were convinced would be proven superior.

After three months of using either the Buteyko or conventional treatments, the subjects were re-evaluated for their use of bronchodilators and steroids and the frequency and duration of attacks. The doctors' confidence in their traditional treatment was shattered when they saw that the Buteyko method helped <u>90 percent of asthma patients reduce or eliminate their use of bronchodilators—while the control group increased use by 9 percent.</u>[2]

Subjects in the Buteyko group also decreased their use of steroids by 49 percent, while the control group showed no change in their use of the drugs. Overall asthma symptoms were also significantly relieved for those following the Buteyko method, with 71 percent showing an improvement in symptom occurrence. Only 14 percent in the control group showed reduced symptoms. A follow-up eight months later revealed that the Buteyko patients continued to get the same level of relief without drugs as they had at the end of the three-month study.

Easy enough for a three-year-old to master

To test Dr. Buteyko's methods, the Medical Institute of E.M. Sechenov in Russia approved a study involving 52 children ages three to 15.[3] All of them had suffered with asthma, some for as long as five years.

Before learning the Buteyko method, all of the children had to use pharmaceuticals, either regularly or intermittently, for asthma attacks or asthma-related problems. Most were selected for the study because their extensive use of drugs had not improved their health or reduced their asthma attacks. Only 10 percent had never been hospitalized, while 90 percent were regular hospital patients.

Patients were given daily instruction for seven days and practiced the Buteyko breathing lessons on their own time to reinforce their instruction. The Buteyko method was so easy and intuitive that most subjects mastered the basic breathing lessons within five to 10 minutes!

The patients were told they could start taking their medications if they were unable to stop an asthma attack after 10 to 15 minutes. For the few subjects who continued to depend on these drugs, their use was reduced by 200-300 percent.

An astounding *73 percent of the children discontinued all use of medications the moment they started the Buteyko breathing lessons.* Of the remainder, 15 percent decreased their use of drugs after three to four days.

Your body will also have to adjust to correct breathing

The foundation of the Buteyko method is learning to breathe through the nose instead of the mouth. To do so, students are walked through a series of short exercises all focused on measured, slow breathing.

While the method doesn't include the use of drugs, there *are* possible side effects. Since your body has to adjust for different-but correct-levels of oxygen and CO_2, it will have to change some of its functions and defense mechanisms. Part of this process is a self-cleansing procedure associated with purging excess mucus, accumulated toxins, and pathogenic microbes from the body. Dr. Buteyko found that these cleansing reactions generally occur two or three times and last from several hours to two days. Some of the reactions include the following:

- Nervous excitement
- Chills and/or raised temperature
- Headaches
- Muscular, intestinal, and chest pains
- Weakness
- Hypersecretion of mucus
- Appetite loss
- Nausea and vomiting
- Thirst
- Excessive salivation when smelling medication
- Increased urination and defecation

92,000 Russians are asthma-free...thanks to Buteyko

Dr. Buteyko's breathing methods have been widely used in the former-Soviet Union and Russia, where it has been proven 92 percent successful in treating asthma. Over 100,000 Russians have been treated with this therapy, and 92,000 of them continue to be free of all asthma medications.[4]

Asthma sufferers, regardless of age, can benefit from the Buteyko method.[5] From mild to severe, asthmatic attacks can be squelched almost as quick as they happen. Better yet, they can be prevented from occurring in the first place—because the method actually eliminates the *cause* of the disease.

While there are practitioners and clinics that teach Buteyko breathing lessons, they are few and far between. And they usually charge $400-$500 per person for the course. Fortunately, you can get all the same information taught in these courses for a lot less money by ordering the Buteyko Home Education Kit. The kit includes a video, a manual, and a workbook—everything you need to learn the method. The 60-minute video is VHS format and even includes a section on teaching the Buteyko method to children. For ordering information see the Source Directory starting on page 213.

If you're under a doctor's care for any health problems, you should let him know that you're planning to use the Buteyko method. The changes in your breathing patterns may reduce your medication requirements—and possibly eliminate them altogether.

References
[1] Med J Aust, 174(2):72-4, 2001
[2] Med J Aust, 169(11):575-8, 1998
[3] www.wt.com.au/_pkold/clinical.htm
[4] www.breathconnection.com/faq.htm
[5] J Asthma, 37(7):557-64, 2000

CHAPTER 13

Serrapeptase:

The silkworm's secret: Ease inflammation and respiratory illness with this enzyme

At some point or another, you've probably seen a nature film showing a caterpillar turn into a butterfly: It weaves a cocoon around itself, and eventually it breaks through the hardened chrysalis, having sprouted wings and changed form almost completely. In the case of the silkworm, there is a specific enzyme called serrapeptase that helps break down the cocoon, letting the newly-transformed moth emerge.

Serrapeptase works by dissolving non-living tissue. This ability captivated researchers around the world, who have subsequently studied its effects in the human body. Some of the claims made about serrapeptase (also known as serratia peptidase) may be stretching it just a tad—we've heard reports that it helps with rheumatoid arthritis, ulcerative colitis, psoriasis, uveitis (eye inflammation), allergies, and may even help fight some forms of cancer. While some of those claims make sense logically, we haven't found enough clinical evidence just yet to tell if they're valid.

But many studies do verify serrapeptase's ability to perform two key functions: it dissolves dead tissue and reduces inflammation. And those functions can ease numerous medical conditions. In human trials overseas, people using serrapeptase have found relief from inflammation, carpal tunnel syndrome, bronchitis, sinusitis, and other ear, nose and throat ailments. According to one alternative medicine practitioner in Germany, it may even dissolve arterial plaque.

Surgical patients treated with serrapeptase experience rapid reduction of swelling

In Europe and Japan, clinical studies have shown that serrapeptase induces anti-inflammatory activity, anti-edemic activity (the lessening of fluid retention), and fibrinolytic activity (the dissolution of protein buildups).[1] Consequently, physicians and patients in Japan, Germany and elsewhere around Europe have begun taking serrapeptase to ease inflammation.

In a multi-center study involving 174 patients, Japanese researchers tested serrapeptase's ability to ease post-operative swelling. One day prior to surgery, 88 of the patients received three oral doses of 10 milligrams of serrapeptase. The evening following surgery, they received one dose. Then for the next five days, they received three doses per day. The other 86 patients received placebos. The researchers reported that "the degree of swelling in the serrapeptase-treated patients was significantly less than the placebo-treated patients at every point of observation after operation up to the 5th day." None of the patients reported any adverse side effects.[2]

Another study involved 66 patients undergoing surgery for torn ankle ligaments. Patients treated with serrapeptase experienced a 50 percent decrease in swelling just three days after surgery. The remaining patients (treated with bed rest, leg elevation, and application of ice in some cases)

ENZYME MAY REMEDY HARDENED ARTERIES

Plaque is the semi-hardened accumulation of cholesterol, calcium, fibrin, and cellular waste products on the inner lining of blood vessels. As you probably know, a buildup of plaque can lead to arteriosclerosis, reduced mobility, blood clots, and even heart attack or stroke.

Hans Neiper, M.D.—a prominent alternative medicine internist from Hannover, Germany—used serrapeptase as part of a treatment protocol to clear plaque from his patients' hardened arteries.

Dr. Neiper began recommending that some of his patients scheduled for bypass surgery should take a combination of serrapeptase and several other natural substances, including magnesium oratate, bromelain, L-carnitine, vitamin B1, and selenium.

Since arterial plaque is non-living tissue, and dissolving non-living tissue is one of serrapeptase's specialties, it may seem like a logical

---

had no reduction in swelling over the same period.[3]

As a note of caution, you should be very careful using serrapeptase or any other anti-inflammatory after surgery until you're no longer at risk for post-operative bleeding. Anti-inflammatories can increase the risk of bleeding, so it's best to avoid using them until your physician gives you the O.K.

Ease respiratory disease in three to four days

In addition to serrapeptase's anti-inflammatory aspects, researchers were also intrigued by its ability to dissolve thick, non-living tissue. In our bodies, retention of fluid and protein can cause the formation of dense mucous, which contributes to the congestion of sinusitis, bronchitis, and other respiratory disorders. Actually, retention of fluid causes these same conditions in other mammals, too. As bizarre as it sounds, some of serrapeptase's benefits have been proven on rabbits with bronchitis.

In Japan, researchers gave serrapeptase injections (20 mg/kg) to rabbits

---

ENZYME MAY REMEDY HARDENED ARTERIES...*CONTINUED*

addition to any arteriosclerosis treatment regimen. But convincing an organization to finance a study on a natural silkworm enzyme that can't be patented (i.e. profitable) is easier said than done, so evidence of the treatment's effectiveness remains limited and solely anecdotal.

However, Dr. Neiper claimed that ultrasound examinations of some patients demonstrated that 12 to 18 months of serrapeptase treatment (or less in some cases) could remove blockages from hardened arteries. His files include cases of patients with restored circulation and mobility, one woman who was saved from hand amputation, and one man whose need for bypass surgery was completely eliminated.

A complete description of Dr. Neiper's protocol and observations is available through the Brewer Science Library in Wisconsin (608-647-6513 or www.mwt.net/~drbrewer).

---

suffering from bronchitis. The enzyme thinned the rabbits' mucous and enabled them to expel more from their lungs. Consequently for a period of one to three hours after treatment, the rabbits breathed easier.[4]

If rabbit mucous isn't enough to convince you (or turn you off entirely), researchers in Italy tested the impact of oral serrapeptase on 193 people aged 12 to 77 who were suffering from acute or chronic disorders of the ear, nose or throat. In a multi-center, double-blind, placebo-controlled study, subjects took 30 mg of serrapeptase a day for seven to eight days. "After three to four days' treatment, significant symptom regression was observed in peptidase-treated patients," the researchers reported. In particular, the treatment eased pain, fever, nasal obstruction, difficulty in swallowing, and anosmia (reduced sense of smell).[5]

Serrapeptase knocks out Carpal tunnel and varicose veins 65 percent of the time

Not surprisingly, researchers have also tested serrapeptase's ability to ease other disorders involving inflammation, fluid-retention, and buildup of fibrous tissue. Carpal tunnel syndrome and varicose veins may seem as unrelated as two conditions could get. But as different as they are, symptoms of both have been dramatically reduced using serrapeptase.

The painful symptoms of carpal tunnel syndrome are caused primarily by inflammation. At the SMS Medical College in Jaipur, India, researchers tested serrapeptase on 20 patients with carpal tunnel. After assessing the subjects' conditions, they instructed the patients to take 10 mg of serrapeptase twice a day for six weeks, then return for reassessment. Sixty-five percent of the patients showed significant improvements. No one reported any adverse side effects.[6]

Fluid retention in and around the veins of the legs causes varicose veins. Researchers in Federico, Italy tested serrapeptase on another 20 people with this condition. The patients took two serrapeptase tablets three times a day (for a total daily dosage of 30 mg) for 14 days. The supplement generated good to excellent improvement also in 65 percent of the subjects. It reduced pain in 63.3 percent of cases, fluid buildup in 56.2 percent, abnormal skin redness in 58.3 percent, and nighttime cramps in 52.9 percent.[7]

Few participants in clinical trials have reported suffering any side effects from serrapeptase. In the varicose vein study, one patient experienced diarrhea, which was alleviated by temporarily decreasing the daily dosage. In other trials, there have been at least two reported cases of serrapeptase-induced pneumonia. However, patients in both cases fully recovered.

Serrapeptase is a blood-thinning agent. Consequently, it may impact anticoagulant therapy and other medications. To avoid any potential complications, consult your doctor before taking serrapeptase. For ordering information see the Source Directory starting on page 213.

References

[1] J Int Med Res 1990; 18(5): 379-88

[2] Pharmatherapeutica 1984: 3(8): 526-30

[3] Fortachr Med, 1989 Feb 10: 107(4): 71-2

[4] Arzneimittelforschung 1982; 32: 374-8

[5] J Int Med Res 1990; 18(5): 379-88

[6] J Assoc Physicians India 1999 Dec; 47(12): 170-2

[7] Minerva Cardioangiol 1996 Oct; 44(10): 515-24

Super Immunity Boosters

Our bodies suffer a constant assault from an ever-growing number of environmental and biological threats. The immune system is our first line of defense against these foreign invaders and infectious organisms. But we are left vulnerable when our natural immune response becomes depressed by factors like drug resistant bacteria, high stress levels, industrial chemicals, environmental pollutants, and nutrient-depleted foods. Our best defense is to develop disease resistance at a cellular level—to strengthen our immune system at the most basic level allowing it to fight off everything from the common cold, to the herpes virus, to cancer.

In this section you will learn about a new product that focuses on skin as the weakest link in your immune system. You will read about the Scandinavian secret to warding off the common cold. You will discover a botanical combination, based on Native American remedies, that researchers are finding is surprisingly effective in fighting off the virus that causes painful cold sore and shingle outbreaks. And you will learn about a Traditional Chinese Medicine approach to conquering stress.

CellAid:

New product focuses on skin as the weak link in your immune system and can help you build up immunity to some of today's most deadly disease

At the Health Sciences Institute, members and affiliates of our international network regularly send us information on breakthroughs for everything from preventing cancer to fighting headaches. Just when we think we've seen everything, something comes across our desks that makes us take a long second look.

Over the years, we've featured several products designed to help you build a stronger immune system, the first line of defense in fighting most diseases. What makes this product, CellAid, so different is the part of your body it focuses on—your skin—and how that can help you build up immunity to some of today's most deadly diseases.

When your skin is in top shape, it can help your liver, thymus, and other immune components fight illness. When it's not, you may be leaving yourself open to infection and even life-threatening microbes. Researchers have discovered that closing the skin's disease-fighting gaps, which are too frequently overlooked, may be a major way to level the playing field against infectious diseases.

Bolstering your skin can recharge your ability to fight disease

There are three main ways your skin helps fight disease. The first is with antibacterial peptides, which neutralize deadly organisms that come in contact with the skin and may protect you from bacterial invasion.[1]

Another important role of skin is to provide a home for T-cells, which are the "foot soldiers" of your immune system in the fight against disease.

In fact, half your circulating T-cells are located in the skin's epidermis. Keeping your skin healthy helps maintain your T-cells' ability to fight illness and aids the maturation process of some immune cells.

Your skin also regulates skin-cell turnover. Proper cell turnover means dead cells are being replaced by new ones at the correct rate. If the replacement process goes awry, cell replacement may become overactive or underactive. Overactive turnover means too many new cells are being made and can result in conditions like psoriasis. Underactive turnover occurs when cells are dying faster than they can be replaced. Either one of these conditions can preoccupy your immune system and prevent it from properly combating infections or other health problems.

Nutrients that target the skin and are specific to its immune system tasks may be able to strengthen your ability to fight disease, but it can be difficult to get enough through food. But now, researchers have discovered a way to use plant-based products that augment the body's cytokines. Cytokines are proteins that are part of the immune system and help prevent the spread of invading organisms.

Nourishing skin for fighting disease requires more than just beauty creams

Most skin-care products, such as emollients, wrinkle removers, and sunblocks, temporarily improve the skin's appearance but usually don't nurture the skin's immune response. Products containing nutrients, such as vitamins A, C, and E, may help repair skin damage, but they may not boost or increase immune cells.

CellAid, a product used for the past 10 years in Europe and the Middle East has just become available in the United States. It's a three-part system containing an oral liquid and two topical creams that helps the skin (and the entire body) in its immune-system duties.

CellAid shows "complete inhibition" of a cancer-causing virus

An independent in vitro analysis conducted by University of California biochemist Kathleen S. Hall, Ph.D., found that CellAid shows "complete HPV-11 inhibition."[2] Human papilloma virus (HPV) is most frequently associated with cancers of the cervix. It is, however, also implicated in other types of cancers, especially those affecting the head and neck area. If you have HPV in your mouth, your risk of getting oral cancer is up to 4.7 times greater.[3] HPV has also been associated with cancers of the lung,[4] sinus cavity,[5] and nasal area.[6]

Increase your body's natural tumor killers

CellAid contains significant amounts of interleukin-12 (IL-12), an important tumor fighter, according to Aristo Vojdani, Ph.D., M.T., of Immunosciences Lab, who conducted an independent chemical analysis of the constituents.[7] Dr. Vojdani claims that raising your levels of this substance may increase your resistance to infectious diseases, spur the activity of your natural killer cells, and stimulate production of your T-cells. Dr. Vojdani also identified a number of other types of immune reinforcers in CellAid, including IL-1a, IL-1b, IL-2, IL-4, IL-5, IL-6, IL-10, interferon-alpha and gamma, and TNF alpha (tumor necrosis factor), and TGF beta (transforming growth factor). This appears to be the first time these cytokine-like immune proteins have been extracted from a plant-based product.

Rasha Yousef Khalil, professor of immunology and head of the immuno-genetic and transplantation unit at the Ain Shams University Specialized Hospital in Cairo, found that CellAid increases the initial immune response by up to 306 percent![8]

This three-part synergistic program may help protect you from serious diseases

To be honest, using CellAid seems a little daunting at first. And if you're someone who can't remember to take your vitamins every day, it may not be for you. Unlike other immune boosters, CellAid is a complete system that must be used together. The liquid is taken and the creams are applied every morning and evening. It is essential that all three components be used to achieve the synergistic effect.

Although this is not as quick as swallowing a few pills, it takes just a couple of minutes to go through the entire regimen.

The liquid, which has a mild licorice flavor, contains 12 active ingredients, including herbal extracts like ginger root, clove buds, cinnamon bark, and hibiscus flower. It also contains fenugreek seeds, which have anti-inflammatory properties and are shown to produce 70 percent inhibition of tumor-cell growth in animals.[9]

One teaspoonful is taken twice a day on an empty stomach 30 minutes before eating. Hold the liquid in your mouth for one minute before swallowing, allowing the cells in your mouth to absorb the nutrients and thereby get a jump-start on delivering them to your bloodstream.

The topical ointments—Skintrinsic SkinGel and Antioxidant SkinSerum— are used alternately. SkinGel contains, among other things, echinacea and panthenol. For the first three weeks, a dime-size portion of SkinGel is applied twice a day, at the same time you take the liquid. Rub in the cream gently and wait for it to absorb, which can take 10-15 minutes.

After the first three weeks, switch from SkinGel to SkinSerum. SkinSerum contains 16 ingredients, including inositol, lipoic acid, maritime pine, and quercetin. Apply the SkinSerum for one week, following the same procedure mentioned above for SkinGel.

The manufacturer suggests using CellAid for a minimum of three and up to six months to help build up your body's immune response. They also recommend taking a two-week break from the product every three months, which will allow your body to continue responding to the formulation instead of becoming used to it. After the initial six-month period, you can use CellAid three or four months throughout the year or whenever your immune system is low, such as during times of illness or stress.

One of the most important factors in supplement use is knowing whether the product is working. Some people may experience temporary immune responses in the first month they take CellAid. These responses, if they occur, are a normal sign of immune system balancing and usually go away after a week or two. Such responses may include a rise in body temperature, fatigue, or an increase of discomfort in areas of pre-existing pain or inflammation. If the response feels too strong for you, simply decrease the amount of CellAid, or stop taking it for a few days.

In some people with high blood platelet counts, high blood pressure, or hyperthyroidism, CellAid may elevate these conditions. This response is usually temporary and the body adjusts. However, if you have any of these conditions, you should be monitored by your doctor and should initially take CellAid only every two to three days (and in lesser amounts than indicated). If you are diabetic or on blood thinning medications (including regular aspirin therapy), you should have your blood monitored regularly as the medication may need adjustment. And, again, please work closely with your physician.

CellAid is not cheap. It's available from Herba-ceuticals only as a complete system, so its components cannot be purchased separately. In order to follow the manufacturer's recommended three to six month treatment regime, an initial investment anywhere from $297 to $594 is necessary. Of course, if you've been battling illness and unable to strengthen your immune system enough to fight it, this could be the solution you've been seeking. For additional ordering information see the Source Directory on page 213.

References

[1] Nord Med, 111(6): 176-9, 1996

[2] Personal communication from Kathleen S. Hall, Ph.D., Univeristy of California Davis, Oct 26, 1998

[3] Oral Surg Oral Med Pathol Oral Radiol Endod, 91(6):622-35, 2001

[4] Histopathology, 38(4):355-67, 2001

[5] Laryngoscope, 111(6):1,104-10, 2001

[6] Head Neck, 21(1):21-9, 1999

[7] Personal Communication from Aristo Vojdani, Ph.D., M.T., Sept. 8, 2000

[8] Personal Communication from Professor Rasha Yousef Khalil, Ain Shams University Specialized Hospital, Oct. 29, 1996

[9] Phytother Res, 15(3):257, 2001

CHAPTER 15

Kan Jang:
The Scandinavian secret to cutting colds by 50 percent

You've got that sniffling, sneezing, coughing, headachy, "just go lie on the couch and suffer" feeling again. And that creates a treatment dilemma for a lot of people. You can take popular cold medications, but they don't always provide adequate relief. You can take antibiotics, but ultimately that helps breed drug-resistant bacteria. So the Health Sciences Institute has researched a natural cold remedy/preventive that promises to be an effective alternative.

Andrographis paniculata, a shrub extract commonly referred to as Indian Echinacea, has been used for centuries in Ayurvedic (traditional Indian) therapies and Traditional Chinese Medicine to treat everything from isolated cases of the sniffles to full-blown outbreaks of influenza. It was credited with halting the spread of disease during the 1919 Indian flu epidemic. More recently, andrographis (under the brand name Kan Jang®) has outsold all other cold medications in Scandinavia for 12 years running. It was named Product of the Year by the Swedish Association of Health Food Producers. And researchers have accumulated considerable data documenting its effectiveness.

Asian herbal extract strengthens your immune system

Andrographis is not an antimicrobial agent. It does not kill the organisms that make you sick—at least not directly. Instead, it boosts your immune system and stimulates your natural antibodies.[1]

Your body makes some very powerful disease-fighting enzymes. If you become ill easily or don't recover quickly from colds and the flu, it's possible that your production of these antioxidant enzymes has been compromised. Andrographis protects those enzymes[2] and consequently enhances your natural disease-fighting ability.

Recover faster and reduce your colds by 50 percent

Chilean doctors tested the effectiveness of andrographis in a three-month, randomized, double-blind, placebo-controlled study in a rural school. Fifty-four students received either two placebo pills or two Kan Jang tablets every day for three months. (Each Kan Jang tablet contains 300 mg of andrographis and no other cold-fighting agents.) A clinician evaluated the students each week to determine if they had symptoms of the common cold. Over the course of the three-month study, **62 percent of the placebo group got colds, while only 30 percent of the Kan Jang group got sick**. Researchers concluded, "Kan Jang tablets have a preventive effect against common colds."[3]

Scientists at the University of Chile in Santiago conducted a larger study involving 158 adults. It was also a placebo-controlled, double-blind, randomized clinical trial, but it was administered for just five days to determine if Kan Jang could help patients recover more quickly from colds. Patients suffering from cold symptoms took either four placebo pills or four Kan Jang tablets a day (a total of 1,200 mg of andrographis daily), and did a self-evaluation of their symptoms at the beginning of the study, after day two, and again after day four. Researchers reported the Kan Jang group experienced a significant decrease in intensity of symptoms (especially fatigue, sleeplessness, sore throat, and nasal secretion) by day two. By day four, they experienced a significant decrease in all symptoms. The researchers concluded that Kan Jang "had a high degree of effectiveness."[4] They also noted that no participants experienced adverse effects from taking four tablets a day.

Meanwhile, doctors in the Hallehalsan Clinic in Sweden conducted two trials of Kan Jang. They found that cold sufferers experienced significant relief from "throat symptoms" after taking the herbal medication. Even though one of the studies treated patients for only three days, doctors saw "highly significant improvement."[5]

Kan Jang reaches maximum potency within two hours

One criticism of herbal treatments is that it often takes a long period of supplementation to generate a benefit. Antibiotics and other prescription drugs work much faster. But, of course, they can also generate some unwanted effects, such as killing beneficial bacteria and creating stronger, disease-causing organisms.

Andrographis is different from most herbal supplements. It reaches maximum levels in the bloodstream 1.5 to 2 hours after it is ingested. Andrographolide, which is the active constituent of andrographis, is "quickly and almost completely absorbed into the blood," according to researchers conducting animal tests at the Guelbenkian Research and Drug Quality Control Laboratory of ADMTA in Yerevan, Armenia.[6] Andrographolide doesn't remain in the body for extended periods of time, which may account for its lack of harmful side effects. According to some researchers, 80 percent of andrographolides are removed via the kidneys and gastrointestinal tract within eight hours, and approximately 90 percent is eliminated within 48 hours.[7]

Andrographis shows other medicinal properties

Andrographis appears to do more than bolster your disease-fighting enzymes. Researchers at the Tongi Medical University in China found the herb can prevent *myocardial ischemia* (inadequate blood circulation in the heart usually due to coronary artery disease) in dogs,[8] while scientists at the National University in Singapore discovered that diabetic lab animals treated with andrographis developed **lower blood sugar levels**.[9] Research has also shown that andrographis can **lower systolic blood pressure** in lab rats bred to be spontaneously hypertensive.[10] Further research has demonstrated that andrographolide treatment can **prevent decreased liver function** in laboratory rodents which were given drugs that would ordinarily impair liver function.[11] Researchers at Yerevan State Medical University in Armenia also found that andrographis could **inhibit the formation of blood clots**.[12]

Such research is very preliminary and limited to animal experiments at present, so the herb's potential to influence these conditions in humans isn't yet known. Extensive human trials of Kan Jang have only measured the product's impact on cold symptoms and occurrences. Those trials have never identified any adverse side effects. However, you should consult with your health care practitioner before supplementing with Kan Jang, especially if you suffer from high or low blood pressure, a blood-sugar disorder, or vascular problems.

Swedish Herbal Institute, the formulator of Kan Jang, recommends that you take 1 tablet four times daily to fight colds or the flu. If you're suffering from allergy symptoms or have sinus problems, you can also use Kan Jang for relief, but at a reduced dosage of two tablets daily. See the Source Directory starting on page 213 for ordering information.

References

[1] J Nat Prod, 56(7):995-9, 1993

[2] Indian J Exp Biol, 39(1):41-6, 2001

[3] Phytomedicine, 4(2):101-4, 1997

[4] ibid, 6(4):217-23, 1999

[5] ibid, 7(5):341-50, 2000

[6] ibid, 7(5):351-64, 2000

[7] www.altcancer.com/andcan.htm (Chinese Herbal Med, 13(9):33-6, 1982)

[8] Tongi Med Univ, 16(4):193-7, 1996

[9] Clin Exp Pharmacol Physiol, 27(5-6):358-63, 2000

[10] ibid, 23(8):675-8, 1996

[11] Planta Med, 58(2):146-9, 1992

[12] Phytomedicine, 6(1):27-31, 1999

TryptoZen, Suanzaorentang Formula (wild jujube), Relora:
Beat anxiety without Prozac:
Panelist reveals five drug-free stress busters

It wasn't very long ago that you couldn't turn around without hearing or reading something about kava. And, unfortunately, the news was not good.

At the end of 2001, German and Swiss health authorities announced they held kava consumption responsible for more than 30 cases of somewhat-serious liver toxicity—including four cases requiring transplantation and one death. The United Kingdom banned sales of all kava products, and German authorities warned manufacturers that their licenses for marketing kava might be withdrawn. The story spilled over to the United States, and, in December 2001, the Food and Drug Administration (FDA) sent letters to physicians asking them to be on the lookout for kava-related liver problems and to report all findings promptly to their Medwatch program. Then, in March 2002, the FDA issued a consumer advisory, "advising consumers of the potential risk of severe liver injury associated with the use of kava-containing dietary supplements."

You may recall the media frenzy that followed—we sure do. The mainstream was all too happy to report something negative about an herbal remedy—despite the fact that millions of people around the world had been using kava for years to effectively treat their anxiety and sleep disorders—and that the main ingredient in Tylenol caused 114 reported cases of liver damage but was still widely available.

Of course, all the while, "traditional" physicians continued to prescribe diazepam (better known by the brand names Valium and Diastat) and other benzodiazepines like Xanax, Restoril, Ativan, and Klonopin for anxiety and insomnia—man-made drugs, each with a long history of serious side effects.

A closer look at kava's bum wrap

We knew better than to expect fair coverage of the kava situation. So last January, we entered the fray too, as one of the few dissenters in support of kava. Panelist Hyla Cass, M.D., author of *Kava: Nature's Answer to Stress, Anxiety, and Insomnia*, is an expert on this South Pacific herb. We asked Dr. Cass to address the kava controversy in an e-Alert, and she cut through the hysteria and laid out the <u>real</u> story about how to use kava safely and effectively. She pointed out that most of the 30 cases identified by European authorities involved the simultaneous use of kava and alcohol or other substances, including prescription drugs known to poison the liver. She also noted that many mainstream over-the-counter and prescription drugs are *far* more likely than kava to cause liver damage.

Still, Dr. Cass warned that kava should <u>not</u> be used by people with known liver problems or by people taking other drugs that may affect the liver. She also recommended limiting daily use of kava to no more than three months at a time, and discontinuing use if there are any signs of liver toxicity such as severe nausea or jaundice.

Today, the mainstream media isn't really talking about kava anymore. But it is still an issue in the alternative health community, and in many people's minds. Many of our panelists still support the use of kava, and many of our members still use the herb. But we've heard from others who are now wary of kava. They want to know about other safe and natural remedies for anxiety and sleeplessness—remedies that don't cause the dangerous and mind-numbing side effects that often come with prescription drugs like diazepam.

There are several other herbs and natural products that reportedly relieve anxiety, reduce feelings of stress, and improve sleep—all with very low toxicity. In fact, most of the natural remedies we found have been tested directly against diazepam, and were found to be far safer.

A safe, calming alternative that won't slow you down

We learned of the first kava alternative from Dr. Cass herself. Since the negative reports on kava began last year, Dr. Cass has been researching other herbal anti-anxiety remedies—and she believes she's found one that is safe, effective, and based on centuries of traditional herbal medicine.

The main active ingredient is magnolia bark, also known by its Latin name *Magnolia officinalis*. In Traditional Chinese Medicine (TCM), it's known as *Hou Po*, and it can be traced back to ancient texts written somewhere around A.D. 100. Magnolia bark contains diverse phytocompounds, including essential oils, alkaloids, and biphenols. These biphenols, specifically honokiol and magnolol, are believed to be the active ingredients behind magnolia's medicinal value.

The anti-anxiety effects of magnolia bark's biphenols, particularly honokiol, are well documented in modern scientific research. In one animal study, scientists compared the behavior of honokiol- and diazepam-treated mice to that of untreated mice. Their activity level was assessed using maze activities and traction tests. The researchers determined that both honokiol and diazepam treatment resulted in calmer mice. The mice treated with diazepam did experience muscle relaxation but only the mice treated with honokiol did not lose any motor skills or muscle tone. When the mice were taken off of their respective treatments, diazepam-treated mice showed signs of withdrawal, while the honokiol-treated mice showed none. The researchers concluded that "honokiol is less likely than diazepam to induce physical dependence, central depression and amnesia at doses eliciting the anxiolytic [anxiety-reducing] effect."[1]

Another animal trial confirmed these findings. In comparing honokiol's and dizaepam's effects on mice's ability to navigate a maze, researchers wrote: "Honokiol at any dose in both single and repeated administration schedules caused neither change in motor activity nor disruption of traction performance." In contrast, mice given diazepam had difficulty finding their way through the maze and took much longer. In summary, the scientists wrote: "...in contrast to diazepam, honokiol selectively induces an anxiolytic effect with less liability of eliciting motor dysfunction and sedation..."[2]

Dr. Cass located an herbal formula that combines magnolia bark extracts with extracts of *Phellodendron amurense*, another ancient herb used for centuries in TCM. It's called Relora, and it has shown promising results in human trials. In one study of 50 adults, 82 percent agreed that Relora "helps control occasional mild anxiety and the associated symptoms." For ordering information, see the Source Directory starting on page 213.

The Chinese anti-anxiety secret that's hard to say, but easy on your system

In our research, we also came across another herbal ingredient with promising effects against anxiety and sleeplessness. It's wild jujube, an herb that has been used in TCM for centuries. It is also known by the Chinese names sour Chinese date seed or Suan Zao Ren, and by its Latin name *Zizyphus jujuba*. Wild jujube is also the main active ingredient in the TCM formula *suanzaorentang*, which is recommended for insomnia, mental fatigue, and forgetfulness. In recent years, modern research has confirmed the sedative and hypnotic effects of both wild jujube alone and in the suanzaorentang formula.

In one animal study, mice given an oral extract of wild jujube root bark showed "a significant dose-dependent reduction in exploratory behavior and spontaneous motor activity."[3] In a double-blind human trial, participants who took suanzaorentang showed "significant improvement in sleep quality and well being" with no side effects.[4] And when researchers compared the

---

OTHER USES FOR THESE ANXIETY-REDUCING HERBS:

Maybe you don't suffer from anxiety, and you don't have any problem getting a good night's sleep. But these ancient medicinal herbs may still help you with other health issues, from heart health to asthma. According to TCM texts, these herbs can be used to treat a variety of ailments, and modern research backs up many of their claims. For instance, studies show that wild jujube can protect against cerebral stroke[6] and protect the heart by improving HDL/LDL ratios and reducing signs of atherosclerosis.[7] Magnolia bark has been shown effective against bronchial asthma[8], and shows potential against Alzheimer's disease and Parkinson's disease.[9]

---

effects of suanzaorentang with diazepam, here's what they found: In patients with clinically diagnosed anxiety, suanzaorentang was just as effective as diazepam at "improving anxiety and sympathetic symptoms." While they did find that diazepam was more effective at relieving overall tension in the body, suanzaorentang showed better results in improving "daytime psychomotor performance." That's an important distinction, because some of the most common side effects of Valium are drowsiness and dullness of mind—not a state you want to be in during the day. In fact, overall the study found that suanzaorentang caused "less and milder side effects...compared to diazepam."[5]

That's good news, especially for our readers over 65, who would be more prone to Valium's potentially serious side effects. Wild jujube is available in the suanzaorentang formula from TCM suppliers. For ordering information, see the Source Directory starting on page 213.

An old folk remedy turns out to be the real thing

So far, we've talked about herbal alternatives to kava. Now let's talk about something completely different.

Remember how, when you were a small child, your mother would offer you a glass of warm milk to calm you down and help you get to sleep? Well, it seems Mom was on to something.

Scientists at Nancy University in France set out to uncover the science behind this "folk wisdom." They hypothesized that one of the amino acid compounds in milk protein was responsible for milk's calming effects. And in a series of laboratory and animal tests, they confirmed it: The milk peptide $as1$-CnTH eases stress and reduces anxiety just as well as diazepam.

The scientists found that when they injected cows with the isolated $as1$-CnTH peptide, it was taken up by the BDZ site of the GABA receptors on the cerebral cortex membrane—the same receptors that take up benzodiazepines, the family of drugs that includes diazepam.

Then they compared the effects of the peptide against the effects of diazepam in rats. In a series of behavioral tests, rats treated with $as1$-CnTH and rats treated with diazepam exhibited similar behaviors, both demonstrating anti-anxiety effects. The researchers concluded that $as1$-CnTH was as effective as diazepam in easing stress and reducing anxiety. Even better, the researchers reported that $as1$-CnTH "does not trigger any side effects."[10]

You could get your $as1$-CnTH from a glass of warm milk…but now it's even easier to get the calming effects of this milk peptide. This research led to the development of an all-natural product called New Life TryptoZen™, which contains isolated $as1$-CnTH in an easy to swallow capsules. TryptoZen is lactose-free, has no known drug interactions and is not addictive. However, if you are allergic to dairy or casein, you should not take TryptoZen. See the Source Directory starting on page 213 for specific information about obtaining it.

Choose the best—and safest—stress reliever for your needs

The media frenzy about kava may have died down. But the need for safe, natural therapies to reduce anxiety and stress is probably greater than ever. The good news is there are plenty of options available—options that don't threaten your health with serious side effects or your well-being with the risk of dependency. We'll continue to search for more natural alternatives and bring them to you through the HSI newsletter and the free HSI e-Alert. For information on joining HSI see page 223 and for information on signing up for the free HSI e-Alert service see page 225.

References

1. J Pharm Pharmacol, 51(1): 97-103, 1999
2. J Pharm Pharmacol, 50(7): 819-826, 1998
3. Ethnopharmacol, 79(1): 13-6, 2002
4. Clin Therapeut, 7: 335, 1985
5. International Journal of Clinical Pharm, Ther and Toxicol, 24(12): 646-650, 1986
6. Chung Kuo Chung Yao Tsa Chih, 21(2): 110-112, 1996
7. Chung Kuo Chung Yao Tsa Chih, 14(7): 434-451, 1989
8. Planta Med, 66(7): 607-11, 2000
9. Am J Chin Med, 28: 379-385, 2000
10. Federation of American Societies for Experimental Biology Journal, 15: 1,780-1,782 1, 2001

ViraMedx and Shingle-EEZE:
From cold sores to shingles:
Control some herpes outbreaks within hours and prevent others entirely

While researching HSI's report on natural treatments for skin diseases we stumbled across a story that was too long to tell in the report and too good not to tell at all. It's the story of how a microbiologist mixed her scientific training with her Native American roots and came up with a unique remedy that is proving to be effective against cold sores, shingles lesions, and other varieties of the herpes virus.

Herpes may not be life-threatening, but it can make you miserable. Then, to make matters worse, it can come back to make you miserable over and over again.

If you get cold sores, you've got company. Between 50 and 80 percent of the U.S. population is infected with the herpes simplex virus, type 1 (HSV-1), which causes cold sores and fever blisters around the lips and inside the mouth. And about one in four adults has herpes simplex virus, type 2 (HSV-2). In addition to painful genital lesions, the symptoms of HSV-2 can include rash, itchiness, fever, muscle aches or a burning feeling during urination.

Perhaps the worst aspect of these viruses is that once you have them, you have them for life. Both remain latent in your nerve cells until they're triggered by any one of a number of factors—for example, a cold or fever, fatigue, stress, or even sun exposure.

Herpes doesn't have to mean a life sentence of painful problems—real relief comes naturally

And while most of us think of the two scenarios above when we hear herpes, that's just the beginning of the effects it can have on your body. If you're over 50, you may be at risk of having herpes zoster. It's the same virus that gave you chickenpox as a child. After lying dormant in your body for decades, it can reemerge as shingles—an extremely painful and persistent disease. Whatever your age, you can develop herpes keratitis, a painful eye infection that produces discharge, light sensitivity, and a gritty sensation in the eye. If it isn't properly treated, it can permanently scar the cornea. In a few cases, a herpes virus can even lodge in the joints, causing intense pain, numbness and difficulty walking.

Simply put, there's no cure for herpes. And mainstream treatments are far from ideal. The leading drug, acyclovir, takes three to seven days to become effective and can trigger severe side effects, including liver and kidney damage. What's worse, it may not produce any relief at all, because several strains of herpes viruses are now acyclovir-resistant.

So we were intrigued when we discovered Viracea, an organic treatment for herpes. And the story got even better when we phoned Meryl Squires of Merix Health Care Products, who developed and patented the formula.

An "Einstein nap" leads to an ingenious herpes breakthrough

Her quest for a cold sore remedy began in her 30s, after she contracted HSV-1. She had a cold sore nearly every month—and they were nasty ones, taking 10-12 days to heal and making her whole face swell.

Reluctant to try acyclovir, Squires drew upon her training in biomedical research and microbiology, and her Native American heritage. Part Powhatan and part Cherokee, she had grown up in a family familiar with natural remedies. For a year and a half, she tested extracts from 52 botanicals and combinations of extracts on herself and accommodating friends and relatives. "Nothing worked! I was so very, very frustrated," she said. She tried botanicals with a track record of fighting herpes, but even potent anti-viral agents like lysine produced disappointing results when applied to cold sores.

One day, discouraged by her research, Squires decided to take an "Einstein nap." It's a technique that Albert Einstein used when he hit a roadblock in his research. He'd focus on the scientific question that was stumping him, then nap for 20 to 30 minutes, letting his subconscious run with it. When he woke, he often had new insights and a key to a solution. When Meryl Squires woke, her first thought was of an anti-microbial (benzalkonium chloride) that her mother used to treat wounds. She wondered if she could produce an effective treatment by combining it with extracts from echinacea and other members of the asteracea family. She prepared a solution and tested it on the cold sore on her lip. "It worked so well it was scary! I really thought it was a fluke."

So she kept testing it…on herself, friends, family, even her horses. (She says it proved to be an excellent treatment for horse herpes and muzzle warts.) All told, Squires spent nine years refining her remedy to the point that she could begin marketing it under the name of Viracea. Then the formal studies began.

ANOTHER POTENT HERPES FORMULA OFFERS 99.7 PERCENT EFFECTIVE RELIEF WITH ABSOLUTELY NO SIDE EFFECTS

Long-time members of HSI will remember that, several years ago, we brought you news about Larreastat, another potent herpes treatment. It's been shown in clinical tests to be 99.7 percent effective for relieving herpes symptoms, with no adverse effects. In dozens of cases, herpes outbreaks were completely resolved within 24 hours.

Larreastat is based on the Larrea bush, a desert shrub used by Native Americans to treat everything from snakebites to digestive problems.

Larrea is rich in nordihydroguaiaretic acid (NDGA) and other phytochemicals with strong antioxidant, anti-inflammatory, antiviral, and antimicrobial properties. It's the antiviral action that makes Larrea a useful weapon against the herpes viruses.

Larreastat is both a topical lotion that can be applied directly to herpes lesions and a nutritional supplement that can be used to help avert impending outbreaks or to speed healing.

Make lesions disappear in less than one day— and even prevent them from forming in the first place

Dr. Ken Thompson, a leading herpes expert at the University of Chicago, exposed 25 strains of the herpes simplex virus and 15 strains of drug-resistant herpes to Viracea in vitro. Although the botanical didn't eradicate the viruses, it was equally effective against both HSV 1 and 2, inhibiting their growth by 50 percent on average. In addition, it was as effective against acyclovir-resistant herpes as it was against strains still susceptible to the drug.[1]

The first small pilot study was promising. Seven people who had tested positive for herpes simplex either sprayed, dabbed, or dropped Viracea on their lesions, then covered the affected area. Over the course of six weeks, they used Viracea on three outbreaks of cold sores and nine of genital herpes. On average, their pain stopped 10 to 20 minutes after treatment; the burning, itching, and irritation ended within four hours, and the lesions dried up and disappeared within 21 hours.

In seven instances, they applied Viracea to what are called "prodrome conditions," symptoms that precede an outbreak of herpes lesions. In all seven, the subjects reported their pain and other symptoms stopped escalating and disappeared within a few hours, and the outbreak of lesions never occurred.[2]

Symptom relief in just five minutes

Next came several large clinical trials. One tested ViraMedx, an ointment preparation of Viracea, on 75 subjects with herpes simplex. Most were carriers of HSV-1, had lesions around their lips, and were suffering from uncomfortable symptoms (including pain, tingling, itching, hypersensitivity, and a burning sensation). After a single dose of ViraMedx was applied topically to their lesions, they reported that their symptoms ceased within five minutes on average; their lesions disappeared within one to 12 days. According to lead researcher Dr. Silvio Boraks, lesions that hadn't yet developed crusts responded much better to treatment.[3]

A larger study involving 300 herpes sufferers—including some with shingles—produced similar results. Symptoms such as pain, tingling, itching, etc., ceased within three to five minutes of treatment; lesions typically healed within one to four days. The most remarkable finding didn't surface until

NATURAL HERPES REMEDY WORKING ITS WAY TO BECOMING AN "ACCEPTED" TREATMENT

Preliminary research and some physicians' reports suggest that Viracea may be effective against several other viruses:

- *human papilloma virus,* or HPV (the virus that causes warts which can lead to cervical cancer and oral cancer);
- *HIV* (Viracea appears to impair the virus's ability to bind to healthy cells);
- *Kaposi's sarcoma* (a form of skin cancer most prevalent among AIDS patients).

Viracea hasn't been tested against any of those conditions in large, formal, clinical trials yet, but the company is pursuing a New Drug Approval from the Food and Drug Administration to have ViraMedx officially sanctioned as a treatment for genital herpes. This is a big step for a natural medicine product.

18 months after the study, however. During follow-ups with study subjects, researchers learned that no one had experienced a herpes recurrence on the area of skin that had been treated with ViraMedx.[4]

As more people tried Viracea products, Merix learned more about their impact on various types of herpes. Shingles sufferers reported that after using Shingle-EEZE (a spray version of Viracea formulated specifically to treat shingles) their pain eased within 30 minutes, their shingles stopped spreading, and, in many cases, existing lesions began to heal within a day and a half. Unfortunately, Merix also learned that Viracea is not effective against postherpetic neuralgia, the excruciating pain that many shingles patients endure long after their lesions vanish.

Medicine goes back to its traditional roots—literally

As Meryl Squires explained to us, "There is a good reason why doctors and scientists did not use traditional medicines in the past. Many weren't standardized and it was hard to determine if they really did work or if they could cause side effects. But now we are bringing those botanical medicines, traditional medicines, back by standardizing them and proving their efficacy so they can be used by the scientific community. It's like we are going back to our roots in traditional medicine."

ViraMedx appears to be very safe. The only reported side effect is a tingling sensation on the treated skin area that lasts a few minutes. There are two precautions you need to be aware of before trying ViraMedx. First, if you're allergic to dandelions or any member of the aster family of plants, you should not use ViraMedx. Second, it's important to confirm that your ailment is actually a herpes virus outbreak before you use ViraMedx. Some outbreaks that look like herpes aren't. For example, yeast infections can generate symptoms that resemble herpes—and not only is ViraMedx ineffective against such infections, it can actually make them worse. Once these two concerns have been addressed, ViraMedx can offer fast, effective relief. For information on ordering ViraMedx or Shingle-EEZE see the Source Directory starting on page 213.

References

[1]   Antiviral Res, 39(1):55-56, 1998 July

[2]   www.viramedx.com

[3]   Clinical Research Study (unpublished) "Experimental clinical protocol of ViraMedx for treatment or oral herpes," Prof. Dr. Silvio Boraks, Instuto do Cancer Arnaldo Viera de Carvalho, Sao Paulo, Brazil, 2001

[4]   Report on Clinical Study of ViraMedx (unpublished) by Prof. Dr. Silvio Boraks, Director of Oral Cancer Dept, Cancer Institute A.V. Carvallo, Sao Paulo, March 11, 2002

Zen:

Amino acid beats stress, protects brain function, and enhances cancer treatment

Stress has been called America's biggest health problem. According to the American Institute of Stress in Yonkers, New York, 43 percent of all American adults suffer adverse health effects due to stress. Between 75 and 90 percent of all visits to primary care physicians are for stress-related complaints and disorders. On any average weekday, one million Americans are absent from work due to stress-related complaints. And stress-induced ailments don't stop with migraines, insomnia, and indigestion. Clinical research has linked stress to all leading causes of death, including heart disease, cancer, lung ailments, accidents, cirrhosis, and suicide.

In Japan—where stress levels are notoriously high and death from over-work is so common that doctors gave it a clinical designation (*karoshi*)— researchers discovered a natural stress fighter in an extract of green tea. *L-theanine* is a neurologically active amino acid capable of inducing chemical changes in the brain that leave a person feeling alert but relaxed. (A rarely occurring amino acid in green tea and some mushrooms, L-theanine is a totally different substance from the more common amino acid *L-threanine*.) Theanine's effect and its taste (a distinctive green-tea flavor called *umami*) became so popular in Japan that the government approved its use in food products (except baby food) and manufacturers developed more than 50 theanine-enriched products, including sodas and chewing gum.

Theanine hasn't been the subject of significant research in the United States and hasn't been used widely in supplements except for the occasional appearance in body-building and sports formulas (due to its reputed ability to stimulate production of human growth hormone). However, research from Japan indicating that theanine can ease stress, protect neural functions, and even enhance cancer treatments is increasing demand for the amino acid in the U.S..

Theanine triggers chemical changes inside the brain

Research on human subjects has revealed that theanine crosses the blood-brain barrier and induces several distinct chemical changes in the brain that reduce an individual's feelings of stress. Approximately 30 minutes after it is ingested, theanine stimulates production of alpha waves. Such brain waves leave a person feeling alert but deeply relaxed. Theanine also stimulates production of gamma aminobutryic acid. GABA, our most widespread neurotransmitter, limits nerve cell activity in those areas of the brain associated with anxiety, and consequently induces a state of relaxation, calmness, and serenity in stressed or agitated individuals.

At the Laboratory of Nutritional Biochemistry at the University of Shizuoka in Japan, researchers found that theanine also "significantly increased" tryptophan,[1] an amino acid that is the basis of serotonin. A mood-altering brain chemical, serotonin is essential to a feeling of well-being and relaxation and may help alleviate symptoms of clinical depression.

Additional research uncovers potential to help stroke and Parkinson's patients

Another University of Shizuoko study indicated that theanine's impact on the brain and nervous system might do more than reduce stress. Researchers found that when theanine was administered to laboratory rats "it caused significant increases in serotonin and/or DA [dopamine] concentrations in the brain."[2] This finding could become important to people suffering from Parkinson's disease. Parkinson's is characterized by a deficiency of dopamine in certain areas of the brain and is commonly treated with L-dopa, a substance that turns into dopamine once it crosses the blood-brain barrier.

In addition to providing the foundation for substances essential to good neuron function, theanine may prevent brain cell death. In a study at Itoen Ltd.'s Central Research Institute in Japan, scientists found that gerbils suffering from induced stroke fared much better if they were pretreated with theanine. One week after suffering a stroke, neuronal death was "significantly prevented"[3] in gerbils pretreated with theanine. The researchers concluded, "These findings indicate that theanine might be useful clinically for preventing

(continued on page 113)

AT-HOME HORMONE TEST REVEALS
PHYSIOLOGICAL IMPACT OF STRESS

Using saliva as a diagnostic tool, researchers have developed a way to measure the physical impact of stress.

Whether it's triggered by bad or good events, stress increases our levels of the hormone cortisol. Although our bodies are well equipped to handle certain amounts of stress, constant stress over an extended period of time can keep cortisol levels at an excessively high rate. That situation can suppress the immune system and lead to stroke, heart attack, infections, and other health problems.

In the 1980s, officials with the international space program realized that astronauts face acute risks of developing stress-related diseases. Consequently, NASA and ESA (the National Aeronautics and Space Administration and the European Space Agency, respectively) contracted Italian scientists with the Interdisciplinary Research for Clinical and Experimental Advancement to devise a method of testing the cortisol levels of astronauts serving on the Mir space station. The test would have to be inexpensive, non-invasive, and free of any need for bulky equipment or time-consuming procedures. The Italians decided against using standard blood tests for serum cortisol levels. Instead, they opted to take oral swabs several times a day and track the astronauts' hormone changes through their saliva.[8]

A conventional blood test can measure an individual's cortisol level at a single, isolated moment. But that reading doesn't provide a complete picture of how stress is affecting a person's hormone levels and health. Cortisol production varies during the day. Typically, it is highest in the morning and wanes as nighttime nears. If you are under a great deal of stress, however, your level can remain high in the evening. By testing your cortisol levels throughout the day, a healthcare practitioner can get a much better idea of how well you are coping with stress and whether excessive cortisol is undermining your health or putting you at risk for serious illnesses.

Following the procedures adopted aboard the Mir station, North Bay Diagnostics of Michigan has produced a simple cortisol testing kit consisting of chewing gum (to stimulate saliva production), four plastic vials, instructions on how and when to collect saliva, and a prepaid mailer to carry the vials back to North Bay's lab. To complete the test, you basically spit into a vial four times over the course of a day. North Bay analyzes the samples and sends back a report that lists the results, compares them to normal levels, and discusses possible health consequences and treatment options. You don't have to go through a doctor to get this test (unless you live in California or New York). However, North Bay's medical director, Chad Kotlarz, N.M.D., recommends individuals should share their results with their physicians in order to obtain appropriate treatment.

See the Source Directory starting on page 213 for information on ordering the cortisol kit.

ischemic neuronal damage." Theoretically, if a substance can prevent the death of brain cells, it may diminish the disabling side effects commonly associated with strokes, increase post-stroke mobility, and reduce rehabilitation time.

Theanine boosts effectiveness of mainstream cancer treatments

While many substances demonstrate only one or two benefits, theanine appears to be much more diverse. Besides having the ability to induce relaxation and protect brain cells, it has been shown to increase the capabilities of mainstream anticancer drugs.

Doxorubicin (DOX) is a drug used to treat tumors. Doctors found that adding theanine to the treatment boosted the potency of DOX by preventing the drug from flowing out of the tumor cells.[4] This allowed DOX to be active longer and potentially destroy more cancer cells.

At the University of Shizuoka School of Pharmaceutical Sciences, researchers found that theanine could even reverse a tumor's resistance to DOX.[5] Although the testing was done on mice bearing leukemia cells, it holds promise for cancer patients who have built up a resistance to mainstream treatments.

In another Japanese study, scientists administered the anticancer antibiotic idarubicin (IDA) to tumor-bearing mice and noted that their counts of white blood cells and bone marrow cells decreased significantly. Administering theanine to the mice, however, "significantly reversed these changes." The scientists concluded that the amino acid "selectively moderates IDA-induced toxicities."[6] Cancer patients undergoing aggressive mainstream treatments often find that their overall health is compromised by the drugs used to fight cancer. Research is still preliminary, but theanine supplementation may be able to combat the depletion of disease-fighting white blood cells and allow bone marrow cells to continue to produce red blood cells.

Because theanine crosses the blood-brain barrier to enhance and protect brain cells, it is important to establish if there is a danger of toxicity at higher levels. Laboratory rats who received high doses of theanine absorbed some of the supplement but still produced high levels of theanine in urine, indicating that excess amounts are eliminated naturally. Significant levels in the blood, liver, and brain were achieved one hour after supplementation, while maximum levels in the brain were seen five hours after taking theanine. Within 24 hours, all traces of theanine had completely disappeared from the tissues of the laboratory animals.[7]

You can get theanine simply by drinking green tea. However, if you prefer not to drink green tea directly, Optimal Health Resources of Florida markets a theanine supplement called Zen. Each capsule contains 100 mg of theanine and 375 mg of GABA (gamma-aminobutyric acid), an amino acid that inhibits the effect of stimulants. For ordering information see the Source Directory starting on page 213.

References

[1] Biosci Biotechnol Biochem, 62(4):816-7, 1998

[2] Neurchem Res, 23(5):667073, 1998

[3] Neurosci Lett, 289(3):189-92, 2000

[4] Toxicol Lett, 121(2):89-96, 2001

[5] Toxicol Lett, 114(1-3):155-62, 2000

[6] Cancer Lett, 158(2):119-24, 2000

[7] Biosci Biotechnol Biochem, 63(4):615-8, 1999

[8] J Gravit Physiol, 5(1):P145-6, 1998

Powerful Pain-relief Solutions

With 48 million of us suffering from chronic pain—pain that lasts for weeks, months, or even years at a time—chances are you, or someone that you know, has been touched by this issue. With conditions ranging from acid reflux disease to migraine headaches many of us find ourselves facing pain on a daily basis. In fact, over 21 million of us are routinely taking prescription painkillers just to make it through the day.

In this section you will find natural and non-addictive breakthrough pain-relief solutions. You will learn about the British compound that has brought blessed relief to many acid reflux and indigestion sufferers. You will discover the traditional Indian herbal medicine that is achieving near miraculous results in treating kidney stones and chronic urinary tract infections. And you will read about a safe, natural, and effective alternative to over-the-counter painkillers for easing pain and inflammation.

Foundation & Renew Formula:
Put alternative medicine's underlying theories to work for you with an amazing natural migraine remedy

Migraine attacks, as you may know, leave people in terrible pain, nauseated and dizzy. What you may not know (we didn't until we started researching this story) is that they're in even greater peril: Migraines are associated with one out of four strokes.

Twenty-four million Americans, most of them women, suffer from migraines. And they're hard to treat. Migraine attacks are triggered by a number of things—medications, food allergies, caffeine, hormones, stress, bright light, loud noises, and more. To complicate things further, medical researchers don't know what causes them in the first place. It may be an imbalance of neurochemicals, rapid cycles of constriction and dilation in cerebral blood vessels, or something entirely different.

This lack of understanding hasn't kept pharmaceutical companies from developing prescription medications and over-the-counter remedies for migraines. Americans alone spend more than $4 billion a year on non-prescription headache drugs. And we get more (or is it less?) than what we pay for. There's a whole boatload of potential side effects, including stomach upset, insomnia, hypotension, rashes, constipation, sexual dysfunction, even liver damage. More immediately, there's the risk of triggering a new attack—a "rebound migraine." Even the prescription drugs don't always work quickly or well enough to get you right back into the swing of your everyday life.

Even alternative medicine fell short for migranes—until now

The alternative health care sector offers a few natural remedies (feverfew, butterbur, and a variety of herbal teas) and recommends supplements (magnesium, vitamin B_2, and 5-hydroxytryptophan) for migraine prevention. And there's always acupuncture. But these alternative approaches don't have consistent documented success in treating migraines, and even less success in eliminating them.

But then Tom Staverosky, a Pennsylvania entrepreneur and natural medicine researcher, stumbled onto something unexpected. He was selling a supplement called Seacure, made of pre-digested fish powder. (It sounds grosser than it is—all it means is that the nutrients have been broken down by enzymes so that you can absorb them more easily.) Seacure had been shown to improve digestion and ease symptoms of Crohn's disease, ulcerative colitis and irritable bowel syndrome.

Unexpected—and beneficial—"side effects" of a natural digestive aid

"There were a handful of doctors who would come up to me at conventions and say, 'I'm getting great results with Crohn's, colitis, irritable bowel, MS, Parkinson's, migraines, and chronic fatigue.' And I thought, 'Whoa, whoa, whoa! Slow down! What is this all about?'"

These accidental benefits ultimately led Staverosky to a dramatically different view of disease and treatment, and a new approach to migraines. Its goal is to return your body to healthy functioning with supplements—and potentially provide a permanent remedy even after you stop using them.

Now, we'll give you fair warning: Staverosky's approach to treatment is not widely embraced by physicians, even alternative physicians. And he bases a lot of it on theory, not on clinical research.

But there's some hard data to support the claims he makes. The data compelled us to take a closer look at the philosophy behind his product—a philosophy that cuts to the heart of alternative medicine.

80 percent of trial participants find partial to near-total migraine relief

While trying to figure out what was going on with Seacure, Staverosky talked with alternative health experts and got a crash course in classic naturopathy. He learned that disease is caused by the deterioration of normal bodily functions. And two of the body's primary functions are digestion (absorbing essential nutrients) and elimination (removing toxins, wastes, and other harmful substances). The basic principle of treatment is simple: If you give the body what it needs, help it eliminate what it can't use, and increase vitality, symptoms will lessen or even disappear.

Working from that theory, he developed an alternative therapy for migraines. It attempts to ease the frequency and severity of migraines by improving the health of the kidneys, liver, and digestive tract. In a three-month clinical trial, 80 percent of participants experienced partial to near-total relief of their migraine symptoms. What's more, Staverosky believes the treatment can reduce the severity and frequency of migraines even after people stop taking it. After witnessing this success, Staverosky's company, Forever Well, introduced a new product to treat migraines.

James Sensenig, N.D., who chairs Forever Well's scientific advisory panel, concedes that not many doctors have embraced the company's approach to migraine treatment yet. But the number of patients reporting relief from their migraines is growing. And, as we mentioned earlier, the treatment's impact has been tested in a formal clinical trial.

Forty volunteers who had suffered from migraines for at least one year and experienced a minimum of two episodes each month tested the product. For three months, they took Forever Well's product which consists of two different components—Foundation Formula and Renew Formula. Participants took three capsules of Foundation Formula and two capsules of Renew Formula 10 minutes before each of their two largest meals of the day. [The dosage for the first three days of treatment was two capsules of Foundation and one capsule of Renew once a day. Then the volunteers took two capsules of Foundation and one of Renew twice a day for the next three days. After those first six days, they switched to the full test dosage. This gradual increase can help to avoid stomach upset and mild digestive problems that may occur.] Participants were not asked to make any other changes in their daily routines. They continued to take other medications as usual, eat their regular diet, etc.

Quality of life increases by 100 percent in just three months

To assess aspects of their health affected by migraines, participants completed a 14-item questionnaire originally developed by pharmaceutical giant Glaxo-Wellcome. The combined quality-of-life score for the group rose from 38 at the beginning of the study to 76 by the end. (It hit 66 by the end of the first 30 days.) Sixty percent of the participants reported almost total relief from migraine attacks. Another 20 percent experienced some relief from the severity and frequency of their attacks. The remaining 20 percent experienced no benefit.[1]

"What I think makes the results even more dramatic," Dr. Sensenig says, "is we didn't do anything about food allergies, we didn't do anything about dietary changes, we didn't stop people from drinking caffeine, we didn't get them to take any physical medicine, any cranial work, anything else. All we had them do is take these two products. So I have to wonder, in the hands of a good alternative practitioner, how much better the results could be."

The hidden connections between your stomach, liver, kidneys, and migraine attacks

The study results are impressive, but still, it's hard to understand how a treatment that improves your gut, liver, and kidneys can alleviate the pain in your head. The answers are theoretical.

Where food sensitivities are involved, the answer seems relatively simple. When you eat a food you're sensitive to, your body fails to digest it properly. Large particles of undigested food leak through the gut wall and into the bloodstream. Your body attacks these "foreign" bodies, and that attack saddles you with allergic reaction. Research shows that improving the health of the digestive tract can boost your body's ability to digest sensitive foods completely. So, theoretically, improving digestion can help ease or prevent allergic reactions like food-triggered migraines.

Similarly, we know the chemicals we absorb through our food, the air, cosmetics, cleaning products and our environment can also trigger or exacerbate migraines. Given that the liver and kidneys are responsible for eliminating toxins and other wastes from our bodies, improving their function could conceivably reduce migraine symptoms.

For hormone-related migraines, the answer is a little more complicated. Dr. Sensenig told me he doesn't have any research or any case studies to show how the Forever Well products could help with migraines associated

(continued on page 122)

HAS ALTERNATIVE MEDICINE LOST ITS WAY?

The world of alternative and natural medicine is being flooded with "a lot of green allopath." At least that's Tom Staverosky's opinion. But to most of us, that phrase doesn't mean a whole lot. Here's how he explained it to me:

He claims that alternative physicians and supplement developers, in order to gain acceptance among mainstream doctors and consumers, have embraced an "allopathic" approach to treatment. In other words, they've tried to present their natural products as specific treatments for specific symptoms.

"Alternative medicine has accepted the double-blind, placebo-controlled study as the gold standard. And while it has its value, it has its unacknowledged limitations. And one of its biggest limitations is it is most applicable to testing the effect of one thing on one other thing. Therefore we have got a lot of alternative research looking at the treatment of symptoms. It's the pharmaceutical model and it is, in my opinion, really hurting alternative medicine."

The pharmaceutical model, Staverosky argues, hides the real potential of natural medicines. For example, it ignores the ability of a digestive aid or a protein supplement to ease a range of chronic ailments simply because doctors and consumers get suspicious if one product promises to do too many things.

"What we are really about is starting to do the kind of work that will get people thinking about what alternative medicine really needs to be," he told me. "It needs to be guided by a different philosophy rather than buying into the existing philosophy."

with menstrual cycles, menopause, or hormone therapy. But he has a theory: Hormone imbalances in the body are the result of one of two conditions—either you're not making the right amount of some hormone or you're not eliminating the right amount. "Hormones," he notes, "are deconjugated in the liver, so improving liver function can affect hormone levels."

Breaking it down: How this breakdown of nutrients helps you

But all this theorizing raises another question. If the key to easing migraines is improving digestion and elimination, why can't you get the same benefit from taking other common digestive aids, such as probiotics, green food products, or other fish protein products?

Theoretically, you can. But Staverosky and Sensenig say their product was designed to be a particularly potent treatment and that the combination of ingredients offers much more benefit than the individual components could. "If you take Seacure, for example, the reported benefits are out of proportion to the amount," Dr. Sensenig says. "You have a 500 mg capsule and the recommended dose is two capsules, three times a day. So you are talking about 3,000 mg of fish. That's a forkful of fish. That's one bite of fish. That's nothing! How could you possibly improve irritable bowel syndrome [or migraines!] with one bite of fish a day? So it seems clear to those of us who have been using these products that the benefits are beyond the nutritional value of the fish."

According to Tom Staverosky, the proprietary fermenting processes used to create Seacure and the ProBio Greens release functional nutrients. The short answer to how it releases those nutrients is simply that the raw material contains a lot of protein. Unfortunately, protein comes in large molecules and large compounds. Your digestive system has to work fairly hard to break down large molecules (which is why it takes your body so long to digest meat) and sometimes (most of the time, actually) it can't completely break them down, so you don't get to absorb all the food's nutrients. The fermentation process uses enzymes to break chemical bonds in the molecules and frees all the nutrients inside. Since they're then smaller molecules, your body absorbs them more easily. (Now if you want the long answer…)

Some of the specific nutrients the fermentation process helps to release are small-chain peptides. Peptides are organic compounds derived from protein that (unlike protein) are easily absorbed by the body. Consequently, they induce a level of healing in the digestive tract, liver, and kidneys that cannot be generated by whole-food products.

Mainstream medicine backs up this view of peptides. There's research documenting that they strengthen the digestive system, facilitate wound healing, and enhance immune response.[2] Pharmaceutical companies have developed intravenous peptide formulas to feed critically ill patients.

Increased energy, healthier skin, and more: benefits way beyond migraine relief

Just like Seacure itself, Forever Well's migraine treatment has some unexpected benefits. And this, once again, brings us back to theory. "One of the interesting things about a naturopathic approach to illness," Dr. Sensenig says, "is that you are not really treating the migraine; you are treating the person's overall functioning. As you improve their health, not only is the migraine going to go away, but any other…illness is going to be affected as well."

As a result, patients taking the Forever Well products reported side benefits ranging from improved digestion and increased energy to better skin (including a lessening of dermatitis symptoms). In addition, Dr. Sensenig told me that Foundation Formula has helped several of his diabetic patients control their blood sugar and even reduce their dependence on insulin (although he's not quite sure why). One patient's blood sugar level dropped dramatically within days after she started on the supplement, making her insulin dose too high. So he strongly cautions that diabetics try the product only under supervision of a doctor and with regular blood sugar monitoring.

According to the developers, no serious side effects have been reported for the Forever Well products. Some individuals have experienced minor digestive problems (diarrhea, constipation); these can be resolved by reducing the dosage or discontinuing use of the product until the problem subsides.

A product with a surprising goal—to get you to <u>stop</u> taking it

Forever Well's migraine treatment isn't designed to be taken long-term. "Our goal is to get you to stop taking our product," says Staverosky . "The concept is that once your body returns to normal function, you shouldn't need us or anything else." The recommended treatment regimen is to take both formulas for three months—and then stop. If the product has sufficiently improved digestion and elimination during that time frame to alleviate the migraines, then the benefits should continue.

A SIMPLE TWO-STEP PROCESS TO MIGRAINE RELIEF— AND BETTER OVERALL HEALTH

Actually, this treatment consists of two separate formulas—one that improves digestion and one that improves elimination.

The Forever Well Foundation Formula (the digestive support) has only two ingredients. The first ingredient is Seacure, the pre-digested fish protein supplement we mentioned earlier. Seacure makes up 75 percent of the Foundation Formula because of its protein content. Protein is critically important to improving digestion and treating nearly all disease. Exclude the percentage of the body that's water, and what's left is 70 to 80 percent protein. Consequently, "if you compromise somebody's protein nutrition, even marginally, almost anything in the body could start to malfunction," Staverosky says. "What I would hear from doctors an awful lot was that 80 percent of the people walking into their offices, regardless of what disease they had, were protein malnourished, not because they weren't eating adequate protein but they weren't digesting or absorbing it properly."

The other ingredient making up the remaining 25 percent of the Foundation Formula is ProBio Greens, a product from New Zealand. It's a mixture of wheat grass, barley grass, alfalfa grass, and spirulina that is also pre-digested using a proprietary fermentation process, which uses enzymes to partially break

---

There's no research to date that measures whether the benefits do persist, or for how long. Staverosky believes they will, as the logical outcome of classic naturopathic treatment. "It is really an individual question," he notes. "But if they eat a relatively good diet and they're not too stressed and they exercise, then the chances are good that the previous symptoms aren't going to come back."

For ordering information on Foundation Formula and Renew Formula see the Source Directory starting on page 213.

A SIMPLE TWO-STEP PROCESS TO MIGRAINE RELIEF...*CONTINUED*

down (pre-digest) the mixture. The edge that this has over other whole-food products is that your body actually absorbs more of the nutrients because the food is already partly broken down.

Combined, Seacure and ProBio Greens provide probiotics, enzymes, and peptides—the three substances most often used to improve digestion.

Once you've laid the foundation, you can begin to renew your health

The second half of the Forever Well equation is called Renew Formula, which combines 21 ingredients that support the proper functioning of the liver and kidneys:

- Eight detoxifying agents, including malic acid, inositol, milk thistle, and celery seed.
- Two antioxidants, proanthocyanidins and superoxide dismutase.
- Ingredients that provide direct nutritional support to the liver and kidneys, such as magnesium aspartate, copper chelate, thiamin, riboflavin, cayenne, beetroot, and Agaricus blazei murill (the potent medicinal mushroom from Brazil that we covered in the May 2002 issue of the HSI Members Alert newsletter. For information on joining HSI see page 223).

References

[1]   Alternative Medicine Review, 6(5): 488-494, 2001

[2]   Townsend Letter for Doctors and Patients, 98-103, 1998 June

C H A P T E R

JointCare:

Ease rheumatoid arthritis pain, preserve joint tissue and mobility–without the side effects of drugs

A medical system practiced in Sri Lanka, India, and Nepal for nearly 4,000 years has yielded an herbal formula that appears more effective than Western medicines at easing pain and preventing tissue damage in people suffering from rheumatoid arthritis.

Unlike other forms of arthritis, rheumatoid arthritis (RA) isn't caused by wear and tear on the joints. Instead, RA is a crippling and still-mysterious autoimmune disease. For reasons that aren't clearly understood, RA prompts the immune system to malfunction and begin attacking healthy tissue, especially cartilage in the joints.

Pharmaceutical companies have developed drugs to ease the joint pain and swelling caused by RA, but those products can induce significant side effects. NSAIDs (non-steroidal anti-inflammatory drugs like aspirin and ibuprofen) can cause stomach pain, bleeding, and ulcers. Cox-2 inhibitors, such as Vioxx, may pose a heightened risk of heart attack. Recently, the pharmaceutical company Centocor issued warnings that its RA drug (an anti-inflammatory called Remicade) could leave users more susceptible to congestive heart failure, tuberculosis, and other potentially fatal infections.

Drug companies have also designed some formulations to slow the progress of the disease. However, nearly all of those drugs include gold compounds which eventually become toxic to the body.

Consequently, most of the nearly 3 million Americans who suffer from RA don't have safe and effective treatment options.

An herbal formulation based on Ayurvedic (traditional Indian) remedies, however, is proving to be **more effective than some conventional arthritis drugs, without the hazardous side effects**.

JointCare from Himalaya USA, the same company that developed GeriCare (profiled in the August 2001 issue of *HSI Members Alert*), is a blend of herbal powders and extracts that have been used in traditional Ayurvedic formulas shown to relieve inflammation. JointCare combines eight herbs that attack both the symptoms of rheumatoid arthritis, as well as the agents that increase inflammation, create pain, and destroy joint tissue.

Ayurvedic formula may stop joint degeneration

At the S.N. Medical College and Hospital in Agra, India, researchers conducted a two-year study of JointCare involving 39 patients. Roughly half of the group received conventional RA treatment, while the other half received JointCare three times daily.

RHEUMATOID ARTHRITIS AFFECTS THE ENTIRE BODY—NOT JUST JOINTS

Arthritis comes in many forms, such as rheumatoid arthritis, osteoarthritis, infectious arthritis, and ankylosing spondylitis (stiffness of the spine). Common symptoms of rheumatoid arthritis go far beyond stiff joints. They include:

- Reduced range of motion
- Fatigue
- Low-grade fever
- Weight loss
- Dryness of eyes and mouth
- Color changes of fingers and toes
- Inflammation of eyes, heart, lungs, skin, or nerves
- Lumps of tissue known as rheumatoid nodules may appear near affected joint (usually near the elbow)

Researchers measured patients' condition, in part, through ESR tests. (ESR is a blood test that indicates the level of inflammation in the body caused by such conditions as rheumatoid arthritis. A high ESR rating indicates a high level of inflammation.) Test subjects in the JointCare group showed an average ESR drop of 52 percent, compared with a 44 percent drop among those receiving conventional therapy.

Before receiving treatment, all patients experienced joint pain. After receiving JointCare three times a day, only 12 percent had joint pain. Meanwhile, 33.3 percent of the conventional treatment group still complained of pain. Stiffness was completely eliminated in patients receiving JointCare, while half the conventional therapy group continued to experience stiffness.[1]

Researchers used one further measure to assess JointCare's potential as an RA treatment. Alpha-I-AT is a protease (an enzyme) that naturally occurs in your body and can prevent diseases like RA from destroying joint tissue. Over the course of the S.N. Medical College study, Alpha-I-AT levels increased by 18.7 percent in the patients treated with JointCare. Levels rose by only 6.1 percent in patients treated with conventional drugs. Consequently, researchers speculate that JointCare may be able to prevent the destruction of some joint tissue and help RA patients retain their mobility.

Numerous other studies have demonstrated that JointCare can effectively reduce pain, swelling, and morning stiffness caused by RA. In one study involving 25 RA patients, 60 percent of the test subjects showed good to excellent improvement in their symptoms after six weeks of treatment with JointCare. No patients reported any adverse side effects.[2]

Another study, published in *Probe* in 1990, followed 17 rheumatoid arthritis patients who were treated with JointCare for periods ranging from five months to two years. All had severe morning stiffness and pain in as many as 12 joints. Patients were taking one or more analgesics and/or anti-inflammatory drugs, and complained of severe gastric problems stemming from this medication. When they began the JointCare study, they were asked to continue their conventional treatment and also take two JointCare tablets three times a day for eight weeks. Researchers conducted weekly checkups to determine if the patients could reduce their dosage of conventional drugs.

"In most of the subjects, it was possible to reduce the dosage without causing any deterioration in symptoms. In two patients, the existing therapy could be completely discontinued and they were maintained on [JointCare] alone."[3]

Possible relief for other types of arthritis

Although RA works differently than other types of arthritis, JointCare seems able to help people struggling with non-rheumatoid varieties of the disease. In 1980, the *Indian Journal of Medicine* published a study of 75

REDUCE YOUR RISK OF RHEUMATOID ARTHRITIS

While medical science doesn't entirely understand the workings of rheumatoid arthritis, it has identified several factors that put people at risk of developing the disease.

A few risk factors are out of your control. For example, women who experienced a short fertility period or suffered previous joint injuries face a greater risk of RA. Likewise, men who were born into a household that used well water stand a greater chance of developing the disease.

But other risk factors are lifestyle choices, and can be modified to reduce your chances of contracting RA.

During a 15-year study of RA sufferers at Linkoping University in Sweden, researchers identified several conditions and lifestyle choices that appeared to increase the risk of developing RA.[8] They include:

- Smoking
- Insulin use (women only)
- Long-term exposure to hair dyes and/or bleach (women only)
- Exposure to farm animals (men only)
- Exposure to household mold (men only)

---

osteoarthritis sufferers ranging in age from 23 to 82. Fifty subjects were treated with JointCare. The remaining 25 served as a control group and received conventional treatment. After nine months of treatment, 40 percent of the JointCare group was pain-free and another 40 percent was experiencing less pain and enjoying an increased range of movement. None of the JointCare patients experienced any gastric problems. Members of the control group experienced short-term or no pain relief.[4]

The formula's active ingredients are:

- Guggul—an anti-inflammatory agent[5]
- Boswellia—fights inflammation[6] and supports healthy joints
- Indian madder—an immune regulator
- Horseradish tree—a stimulant
- Gokshura—a natural steroid that reduces inflammation[7]
- Musk mallow—supports healthy joints
- Guduchi—inhibits bacterial growth and supports the immune system
- Licorice—stimulates the immune system

JointCare is available direct from the importer, Himalaya USA, which is a branch of the manufacturer, The Himalaya Drug Company of Bangalore, India. The recommended dose is one or two capsules daily. For ordering information, see the Source Directory starting on page 213.

References
[1] Antiseptic, 75(5):264, 1982
[2] Rumalaya (Jointcare) Product Monigraph, The Himalaya Drug Company, pp. 23-24
[3] ibid pp. 29-20
[4] ibid pp. 31-32
[5] ibid
[6] Agents Actions, 18(3-4):407-12, 1986
[7] Planta Med, 67(2):196-8, 2001
[8] Ann Rheum Dis, 60(10):934-9, 2001

CHAPTER

Lumbricus Tonic (Earth Dragon):
Earthworms ease pain and upset of Crohn's, colitis, and other bowel diseases

In North America, they're usually consumed only by tequila lovers and eight-year-old boys trying to get a rise out of eight-year-old girls.

In China, Korea, and Vietnam, however, practitioners of Traditional Chinese Medicine (TCM) have used earthworms—powdered, sliced, and occasionally wriggling—in tonics for centuries. And that ancient knowledge has now translated into a 21st century remedy. One physician, trained in both modern Western and traditional Eastern medicine, has developed a formulation of earthworm extract and herbs that may provide relief to chronic sufferers of Crohn's disease, ulcerative colitis, and other inflammatory bowel diseases (IBDs). Over the years, we've covered a number of fascinating breakthroughs. But the history of this therapy has been among the most intriguing.

Identified by their pharmaceutical name Lumbricus (literally, earth dragon), earthworms are used to combat many diseases, including asthma, palsy, and hypertension. (See the box on page 137.) However, research in Asia and North America now indicates that earth dragon is particularly effective in treating intestinal disorders. While we often associate worms with such disorders, we haven't normally viewed worms as the *cure*.

Patients experience complete remission of IBDs

During the second half of the 20th century, mainstream physicians tried to rid every man, woman, child, and beast of worms, because they believed the parasites were a significant cause of disease. However, in Third World countries, where many people have intestinal parasites, cases of inflammatory bowel diseases, such as Crohn's disease and ulcerative colitis, are rare.

University of Iowa professor Joel Weinstock, M.D., a specialist in IBDs, believes the eradication of parasitic worms in developed nations may have actually increased the occurrence of chronic disorders.

Dr. Weinstock and other researchers at the University of Iowa tested a worm treatment on six IBD patients. The subjects suffered from chronic Crohn's disease or ulcerative colitis and had failed to respond to drug therapies. Weinstock gave each a drink containing microscopic eggs from one species of intestinal parasitic worm. The worms would eventually grow to a length

---

INFLAMMATORY BOWEL DISEASES CONTINUE TO BAFFLE RESEARCHERS

Crohn's disease and ulcerative colitis are classified as inflammatory bowel diseases, involving one or more parts of the GI system. They produce several similar symptoms, which can be confusing to patients as well as doctors. They are sometimes referred to collectively as colitis, which confuses things even more. However, there are some significant differences between the two diseases.

Crohn's disease usually affects the lower part of the small intestine, the colon, or both. Symptoms include diarrhea, nausea, severe stomach pain, fever and chills, weakness, and loss of appetite and weight. Mainstream treatments include steroids, antibiotics, and/or surgical removal of the part of the bowel that is causing the symptoms.

Ulcerative colitis is typically an inflammation of the large intestines and rectum. Symptoms include profuse watery diarrhea containing blood, mucus, and pus; rectal spasms; severe intestinal pain; fever and chills; anemia; and weight loss. Mainstream treatments include steroids and anti-inflammatory drugs. If the symptoms are severe enough, surgical removal of the anus, rectum, and colon is performed (in which case the patient is considered "cured").

---

of half an inch. However, they couldn't reproduce and would die off within six months.

Within a few months, all six test subjects experienced relief from their symptoms. Five of the six eventually experienced complete remission of their disease. The fifth required additional worm treatments before going into remission.[1]

But you don't necessarily have to create a colony of living parasites in your intestines to experience the benefits of Lumbricus.

Practitioners of TCM have used powdered earth dragon to relieve IBDs for centuries. Paul Cheney M.D., a researcher in immune disorders, believes both types of worm treatments release the same potent substance. According to Cheney, the peptides (amino acids) in worms appear to provide relief. In an Internet chat forum for the Dallas-Fort Worth Chronic Fatigue Syndrome Support Group, Dr. Cheney noted that a professor at the University of North Carolina treats all his Crohn's patients with earth dragon peptides.[2]

Treat your entire digestive system, not just the symptoms

Mainstream medicine still doesn't know exactly what causes IBDs. Common treatments include harsh, sometimes life-threatening drugs. Glaxo Wellcome's drug Lotronex®, for example, was recalled after five people died and 70 others developed severe side effects, including ruptured bowels and reduced blood flow to the intestines. Other forms of treatment include major surgery in which the "offending" section of the intestine or organ is removed as though it were unaffected by—and had no effect on—the rest of the gastrointestinal (GI) tract.

Even though Crohn's disease and ulcerative colitis appear to have different origins (see the box on page 134), practitioners of Traditional Chinese Medicine believe these diseases are linked to overall dysfunction in the gastrointestinal tract. In fact, some doctors feel that IBDs may be a reaction to a general or overall immune response that has gone awry.[3]

TCM practitioners believe earth dragon has a "tonic effect" on the digestive system that can ease all IBDs. They believe dragon enables the gastrointestinal tract to handle the unique needs and operations of an individual's body, ultimately helping the tract achieve optimal function.

Because earth dragon use has been largely limited to traditional Asian medicine, there are few studies on its effects. The only published articles we found focused on its ability to increase blood circulation and prevent thrombosis (blood clots). Tests at Shanxi Medical College in the People's Republic of China concluded that it lowers aggregation of platelets, "promoting blood circulation to remove stasis."[4] Researchers at Miyazaki Medical College in Japan administered earthworm powder to healthy volunteers, age 28 to 52. After 17 days, the volunteers' blood samples showed an increase in natural anti-clotting agents.[5]

Formula combines earth dragon with traditional healing herbs

Hoang X. Ba, M.D., Ph.D. is a third-generation medical doctor versed in Western medicine and Chinese/Vietnamese herbal therapy. According to Dr. Ba, there have been numerous recent trials in Vietnam that have demonstrated both the safety and efficacy of earth dragon therapy. Dr. Ba says earth dragon treatments have elicited better results than pharmaceuticals in the treatment of a number of serious illnesses, including IBDs.[6]

As a result of his research, Dr. Ba has developed a new formulation that combines earth dragon with three other ingredients that have been used for thousands of years in Asian medicine to treat GI disorders.

Two of the herbs, Acorus gramineus (an antidiarrhea agent) and Poria cocos (used to bolster the power of Acorus gramineus) are found in many TCM formulations intended to prevent gastric problems.[7] Poria cocos was put through 20 years of clinical tests at Henan College of TCM in China. During that time, researchers treated 419 cases of diarrhea with compounds containing the herb. They reported that 96.4 percent of the patients improved and 90 percent were cured.[8] Patients also recovered faster than in studies that tested other herbal preparations or pharmaceuticals. Doctors claimed that Poria cocos' mechanism inhibits germs, normalizes and improves intestinal immunity, accelerates digestion and nutrient absorption, and slows intestinal movement.

The fourth ingredient in Dr. Ba's herbal compound is Atractylodes alba, which is reputed to help speed the healing of inflamed tissues. This herb has such a profound effect on tissue regeneration and the healing process that it is used for recovery from bleeding ulcers.[9] Atractylodes alba helps prevent Candida infestation, or yeast overgrowth, (a common ailment in IBD sufferers) and protects the intestinal tract from further infestation.[10]

There are no independent studies on Dr. Ba's formulation to date. And we fully appreciate that any IBD sufferer has to treat an addition to his diet

---

EARTH DRAGON THERAPY HAS HUNDREDS OF USES

Earth dragon is used in Asia as a fresh medicinal commodity. But you don't have to down a bowl of earthworm soup (a Korean delicacy believed to promote overall good health) in order to feel the benefits of this ancient therapy.

Lumbricus is distributed in powdered form. Earth dragons are harvested in late spring or early summer, cleaned, and dried in the sun. Sometimes, they're even roasted. Only the extract of earth dragon is used in some TCM supplements. In others, the whole earthworm is pulverized and used.

Earth dragons (either as an extract or in whole-pulverized form) have been used traditionally to treat a variety of ailments, including:

- fever, toothaches, ear and throat infections
- chronic hypertension, nervousness, and headaches
- convulsions, seizures, and palsy
- chronic wheezing, bronchial disorders, and asthma
- pain and swelling of joints or stiffness in extremities
- urinary and kidney disorders
- parasites, abdominal distension, and digestive disorders

Earth dragons have also been applied topically to treat burns and skin ulcers

---

with caution. But the history and folklore behind the ingredients in this formula are impressive. And if you suffer the unrelenting pain and discomfort of Crohn's disease, colitis, or some other IBD, it may provide the relief you've been searching for—without the side effects of drugs.

Like most TCM therapies, Dr. Ba's traditional formulation is designed to avoid symptomatic treatment. It aims, instead, to relieve the foundation of inflammatory bowel disease, which is traditionally viewed as an overall GI dysfunction. His proprietary blend of earth dragon, Atractylodes alba, Poria cocos, and Acorus gramineus is available in Lumbricus Tonic, which is sold exclusively by Nutricology, a division of Scottsdale Scientific in Arizona.

Nutricology's Lumbricus Tonic contains 1,500 mg of the four herbs. The recommended dose is three capsules, twice a day between meals. For ordering information see the Source Directory starting on page 213.

References

[1] http://ibd.patientcommunity.com/features/weinstock.cfm?link_id-1786

[2] Chronic Neuroimmune Disease, Paul Cheney, M.D.: Balance the Th1/Th2 Immune System, www.sonic.net/melissak/cheneyis.html

[3] ibid

[4] Zhongguo Zhong xi Yi Jie He Za Zhi, 12(12):710, 741-3, 1992

[5] Southeast Asian J Trop Med Public Health, 23 Suppl 2:131-40, 1992

[6] www.nutricology.com/Newsletter/earthdragon1.htm

[7] Zhongguo Zhong xi Yi Jie He Za Zhi, 9(5):272-3, 1989

[8] Zhongguo Zhong xi Yi Jie He Za Zhi, 11(2):67, 79-82, 1991

[9] Yakugaku Zasshi, 111(1):36-9, 1991

[10] Immunopharmacol Immunotoxicol, 23 Suppl 2:131-40, 1992

Nexrutine™:
Natural version of "super aspirins" stops inflammation, pain...and may prevent ulcers rather than cause them

If you or someone you love suffers from chronic pain, you're likely familiar with the bittersweet relief of pharmaceutical painkillers. For most, it's not much of a choice: either live in excruciating pain or take the drugs so you can get out of bed in the morning—and hope you're able to live in reasonable comfort before they tear your stomach apart. But HSI has learned of a natural, safe alternative to these drugs that may finally give you more of a choice.

NSAIDs—nonsteroidal anti-inflammatories like aspirin and ibuprofen—have proven to be effective painkillers. But they are known to cause stomach upset, ulcers, liver and kidney impairment, and gastrointestinal bleeding. Even the "super aspirins"—COX-2 inhibitors such as Vioxx and Celebrex—reportedly pose a heightened risk of cardiovascular complications, including blood clots, heart attacks, and strokes. In total, more than 260,000 hospitalizations and 26,000 deaths each year are associated with long-term use of anti-inflammatories.

But one company in California believes it may have discovered a safe, natural alternative to over-the-counter painkillers. This substance, called Nexrutine, is derived from an Asian tree and appears to be a botanical variation of the super aspirins. Studies show Nexrutine eases pain and inflammation by preventing the release of cyclooxygenase 2—more commonly known as COX-2—a chemical in the body that causes inflammation and, consequently, pain. But unlike many anti-inflammatories, Nexrutine doesn't cause stomach upset. In fact, it may even prevent the formation of ulcers.

The future of pain relief found in ancient folk remedies

Next Pharmaceuticals—a natural products research and development company based in Irvine, California—began producing Nexrutine following a two-year search for a pain-killing botanical.

After investigating dozens of plants used in folk remedies, Next focused its research on *Phellodendron amurense*—a member of a plant family that has been used in traditional Chinese medicine (TCM) for 1,500 years to treat inflammation, arthritis, and abdominal pain. TCM practitioners refined an extract of the Phellodendron's yellow bark into a drug known as huang-po.[1]

Traditional botanical wisdom (and subsequent laboratory testing) also revealed that Phellodendron contains an alkaloid called berberine that has been used in Ayurvedic, Chinese, and other traditional medicines to kill bacteria and reduce inflammation for at least 3,000 years.[2] Earlier this year, researchers from the faculty of pharmacy at Gazi University in Ankara, Turkey administered an extract containing berberine to mice and rats

---

A PAINKILLER THAT PREVENTS ULCERS?

An ulcer is an area of tissue erosion, often in the lining of the gastrointestinal tract. Most frequently caused by a bacterial infection, ulcers can also be caused or exacerbated by stress, smoking, and anti-inflammatory medications.

In several tests on laboratory rats and mice, Phellodendrun amurense has demonstrated an ability to inhibit the development of ulcers linked to aspirin, ethanol, stress, and other factors. Researchers have concluded that it prevents ulcers in two ways: by protecting cells in the GI tract and by lowering production of gastric acid.[8]

Scientists working for Kampo Research Laboratories in Osaka, Japan, uncovered further evidence of Phellodendron's anti-ulcer abilities. While analyzing the components of a traditional Chinese medicine for ulcers, they determined that oral doses of Phellodendri cortex (ranging from 25 to 100 mg/kg) inhibited the appearance of ethanol-induced lesions in the gastrointestinal tract—often the first phase of a gastric ulcer.[9]

---

suffering from inflammation. They observed "potent anti-inflammatory effects."[3]

Nexrutine eases pain by blocking inflammation before it starts

Convinced that *Phellodendron amurense* was safe for human consumption and held potential as a painkiller, Next began conducting its own clinical research. Pharmacological screening showed that the botanical contains several anti-inflammatory fractions that also appeared to be analgesics (pain relievers). It also revealed that Phellodendron contained a stress-reducing component.

"There is an anxiety component to pain," says Robert Garrison Jr., pharmacist and chairman of Next Pharmaceuticals. "If you can take down the stress component while you're giving an analgesic or anti-inflammatory, you can have better overall pain reduction."

Next combined the stress-reducing fraction with the key anti-inflammatory compound, and began testing the botanical's ability to ease pain.

Researchers at Cerep, a laboratory in France, exposed human cells to agents that trigger a release of COX-2 and then added Nexrutine to the cell culture. The tests showed the extract was 95 percent effective at inhibiting the enzyme's release. Nexrutine, however, functions in a different way than many other COX-2 inhibitors: Rather than inhibiting the enzyme itself, Nexrutine inhibits the gene that triggers production of the enzyme, thus preventing inflammation from happening in the first place.

The researchers then tested Nexrutine's impact on COX-1, an enzyme that helps maintain the lining of the stomach and promotes healthy kidney function. Often, agents that suppress COX-2 expression also suppress COX-1, causing gastrointestinal distress and disease. Nexrutine did not inhibit the release of COX-1, thus not contributing to any gastrointestinal diseases.[4,5]

Study proves natural alternative as effective as popular "extra strength" over-the-counter pain reliever

In tests on laboratory animals, Nexrutine was compared to naproxen (a popular and long-acting NSAID, commonly found in products like Aleve and Naprosyn). Researchers gave each animal two doses of either Nexrutine

(200 mg/kg) or naproxen (100 mg/kg)—one dose was given 70 minutes before administering an inflammation-inducing solution called formalin, the second dose 10 minutes before formalin. Nexrutine proved as effective as naproxen in offsetting inflammation and pain.

In an effort to determine how quickly and how long Nexrutine could treat pain, researchers gave different groups of laboratory animals 200 mg/kg of Nexrutine at different intervals ranging from 10 minutes to five hours before the formalin. The tests showed that Nexrutine acts quickly, significantly easing pain when taken as little as 10 to 30 minutes before the onset of inflammation. And the effects are long lasting—still providing relief when taken as much as three to five hours before inflammation was induced.[6]

In a human trial, researchers asked 53 dietary supplement users to take two to three 250-mg Nexrutine capsules every day for two weeks. All the subjects suffered from joint or muscle pain, but none were taking prescription pain medications. Seventy-two percent of subjects said that Nexrutine effectively relieved stiffness and pain in the muscles and joints and enabled them to engage in more physical activity with less discomfort. No one reported any significant side effects, and 86 percent said that Nexrutine was gentle on their stomachs.[7]

Patients with arthritis and fibromyalgia find relief within seven days

At his clinic in Cincinnati, James LaValle, R.Ph., N.M.D., C.C.N., has used Nexrutine to treat between 150 and 200 patients suffering from arthritis, fibromyalgia, and general joint and muscle pain. On average, the extract has proven to be 70 percent effective at delivering ongoing pain relief, improved mobility, and diminished morning stiffness within seven days of beginning treatment.

A proponent of integrative medicine and author of the book The COX-2 Connection: Natural Breakthrough Treatment for Arthritis, Alzheimer's, and Cancer, Dr. LaValle was particularly interested in finding an anti-inflammatory that didn't carry severe side effects.

"Pain control is important, but I think what is more important is your health," LaValle says. More than 80 percent of Americans over the age of 50 currently suffer from some form of arthritis, and people are developing the disease at younger and younger ages. "So you have people in their 20s now taking drugs that used to be reserved for people in their 50s. What does that say about the longevity of their kidneys and their livers and other vital organs? That's where my concern lies, and that's why I like people looking for safer first options for pain management."

Nexrutine combination formulas: The next arthritis powerhouse

While Nexrutine is currently being combined with other ingredients (such as glucosamine and chondroitin) in several natural pain-relief formulas, you can also buy pure Nexrutine. Recommended dosage is two to three 250-mg capsules daily. Researchers at Springborn Laboratories in Spencer-ville, Ohio, have verified that Nexrutine is not toxic even at much higher doses. They administered a single extreme dose (5,000 mg/kg) to lab rats and found "no significant gross internal findings" when they euthanized and autopsied the animals 14 days later.[10]

While Nexrutine does not appear to cause gastric upset, all NSAIDs and COX-2 inhibitors have the potential to reduce kidney function and increase the risk of high blood pressure. Consequently, Nexrutine should be used with caution. If you suffer from impaired kidney function, heart disease, or hypertension, consult your physician before trying this supplement. See the Source Directory starting on page 213 for ordering details.

References

[1] Oriental Materia Medica: a concise guide, pages 162-163

[2] www.thome.com/altmedrev/fulltext/berb.html

[3] J Ethnopharmacol, Feb 2002; 79(2): 237-48

[4] "Nexrutine Research & Development," Next Pharmceuticals, Inc., November 6, 2001

[5] "Review and opinions on the pharmcological properties of Nexrutine," Kazunori Faduka, M.D., Associate Professor, Department of Oriental Medicine, Gifu University School of Medicine, Japan

[6] "Nexrutine Research & Development, " Next Pharmceuticals, Inc., November 2001

[7] "Nexrutine Human Trial Report," Dennis and Company Research, September 2000

[8] Yakugaku Zasshi 109(9) 1989, pp 672-676

[9] Jpn J Pharmacol 1989 Mar; 49(3): 301-8

[10] "An Acute Oral Toxicity Study in Rat with SAC1-0004X: Final Report," Dawn D. Patterson, B.S., October 17, 2000

Potter's Acidosis:
Relieve acid reflux and indigestion with British compound

We all suffer occasionally from acid indigestion. When it's continuous, however, it's not only painful, it can be dangerous. Acid reflux (which funnels acid up out of your stomach and into your esophagus) can damage esophogial tissue and create even more burning discomfort. And relief is hard to find. Conventional medications often provide an incomplete remedy or carry

---

KICKING OUT THE PURPLE

...BY HSI PANELIST ALLEN SPREEN, M.D.

This is so sorry an issue that it gives me reflux. I can't tell you how many times I've stopped 'heartburn,' 'reflux,' 'acid indigestion,' whatever...now it's called 'GERD' [GastroEsophageal Reflux Disease] to make it really official! If everyone would just give me $1500/year to stop it, I'll pay for the supplements myself and retire a VERY wealthy man with what's left (and improve the patient's digestion at the same time).

The solution is ridiculously simple (and cheap). Using readily available acidophilus and digestive enzymes I stop over 2/3 of all cases. The more difficult cases (that may include overt ulcers, etc.) may involve a more aggressive approach, but omitting really serious GI illness the results are nearly always extremely positive.

'Reflux' (or any of the other scary sounding names) is nothing more than acid slipping past the junction of the stomach and esophagus. The stomach is designed for it, the esophagus is not...hence a trap door (sphincter) at the intersection (called the GE, or GastroEsophageal junction) set in place to keep the two areas separated.

(continued on page 146)

---

unpleasant side effects.

In Great Britain, however, a simple herbal remedy has been providing people with effective, safe, thorough relief of acid indigestion and reflux for more than 100 years. Incredibly, it has not made its way to the United States...until now.

Readers of HSI's e-Alert (for information on signing up for the FREE HSI e-Alert see page 225) may recall our first coverage of this natural cure. See the sidebar, starting on page 145, for a excerpt from that HSI e-Alert.

KICKING OUT THE PURPLE...*CONTINUED*

Acid essentials

People act like (from propaganda on TV) stomach acid is some kind of mistake on mother nature's part. How many times in my practice have I had to repeat that ACID IS SUPPOSED TO BE DOWN THERE...WE NEED IT!

Here's the kicker: if you 'kill it off' (using antacids, acid blockers, etc.) the body, in its wisdom, saves the energy required to protect the esophagus from the stomach's (normally) more acid environment and weakens the GE sphincter. This allows any remaining acid to sometimes slip past and irritate the esophagus. So, you take an antacid (or whatever...we have so many choices these days) and you feel better, because you lessen even more what little acid remains that has been irritating your already sensitive esophagus.

The above association reinforces that you need more antacid next time, since it helps in the short term. So look what's happening—the short term 'fix' assures that the problem will continue (and even worsen).

Is that not the most beautiful trick? The 'cure' assures its own increasing necessity...it's positively brilliant (and diabolical). And don't think for an instant that I'm the only one who's figured it out (and I make no money on the system).

Acidophilus & enzymes

Acidophilus supplements (powder form, the liquid tastes awful) protect the esophagus without killing acid (while killing the pain almost immediately).

Back in December 2001, we related this discovery from panelist Allan Spreen, M.D. after his colleague experienced incredible relief from acid indigestion by using this herbal remedy.

Dan Denning was hounded by acid reflux for years. After trying various over-the-counter drugs, his doctor prescribed Prilosec®—one of the many medications being featured in the flood of TV drug commercials these days. However, like most drug-commercial darlings, Prilosec also comes with its own quick list of side effects—some just an uncomfortable nuisance, some

---

KICKING OUT THE PURPLE...CONTINUED

The hassle is, you have to keep it handy and take it often if you don't solve the whole problem, which involves tightening the GE sphincter. That can be done using the English herbs (Potter's Acidosis) or by improving the environment of the stomach, which then tightens the junction on its own but requires a bit more effort.

When the stomach is low on acid it tends to also be low on digestive enzymes. Believe it or not, the solution (along with acidophilus protection) is to ADD acid and digestive enzymes at the same time. Remember, it isn't acid that's the problem (you need it desperately for digestion); it's acid reaching the esophagus. Proper digestion allows for higher concentration of acid while tightening the GE junction and protecting the esophagus. I do that using Super Enzymes by TwinLab, two capsules at mid-meal. I hate to push just one company, but it's one of the few enzymes that includes betaine hydrochloride, a plant-based form of acid like what's in the stomach (you hope)—plus it's available everywhere. I'm sure there are others.

A trick with acidophilus capsules is that, with reflux, you must open the capsule and let the saliva carry it down the throat to the stomach. Dose is no problem, as the supplement represents a sample of the billions of 'good guy' bacteria that you want in the GI (gastrointestinal) tract (and in which most people are woefully deficient). Look for caps measuring at least 1 billion (with a 'B') cfu (colony forming units).

(continued on page 148)

potentially serious. The list includes headaches, dizziness, skin rashes, diarrhea, vomiting, and stomach pain.

Unhappy with the drug, Dan continued to search for an alternative. On a trip to England, he mentioned his problem to a friend, who told him about Potter's Acidosis—a natural remedy made by a British herbalist in business since 1812.

Fights the source of acid reflux while relieving symptoms

Potter's Acidosis is made from meadowsweet, charcoal, and rhubarb, which have long histories of calming gastrointestinal disorders.

Meadowsweet has been studied extensively and shown to have anti-ulcer

---

KICKING OUT THE PURPLE...*CONTINUED*

Licorice stick

Occasionally the combo of acidophilus and digestive enzymes isn't enough (that's uncommon), or there is actual stomach trouble from low acid (the stomach's defenses weaken over time, too, with decreased acid, such that irritation there can form and progress to an ulcer...see how these things are connected?). Then, I add DGL, a form of licorice that has one component removed (DGL means De-Glycerrhizinated Licorice). I use Enzymatic Therapy brand but there are other good ones. Chewing or sucking on one 20 minutes before eating can be very helpful in difficult cases. Avoiding refined sugar and white flour products also seems to help.

The Potter's solution can be very effective; just bear in mind that it is a 'fix' that does not repair the altered state of the gastric environment.

Killing off acid, however it's done, is a serious mistake with long term consequences if pursued over time. Poor digestion is the genesis of all sorts of problems, in my opinion...but that's just me.

Good Health,

Allan Spreen, MD

---

activity. It can even protect the stomach from lesions associated with aspirin use.[1]

Rhubarb has been used in traditional Chinese medicine for gastric disorders and as a treatment for bleeding duodenal ulcers.[2] It has also been shown to fight bacterial growth in the intestinal tract[3]—an important function in people suffering from digestive disorders, since bacteria can grow in food that isn't properly digested in the stomach.

Charcoal, while not widely known today, has been a mainstay of natural medicine. One of the properties of charcoal is its ability to quell gas in both the stomach and the intestinal tract. When whole or partially digested food is passed through the digestive system, it can cause gas as a side effect. Charcoal often alleviates that problem.

Experience near permanent relief with occasional use

When he first started using Potter's Acidosis, Dan got immediate relief from his acid reflux without any unpleasant side effects. He now takes the supplement only when he has a problem—which is rare.

We have not been able to locate anyone in the United States who sells Potter's Acidosis. However, you can purchase it, using a credit card, from Potter's Herbal Supplies in England. For ordering information see the Source Directory starting on page 213.

Please note: If you are taking blood-thinning medication, check with your doctor before using Potter's Acidosis; meadowsweet contains heparin (an anticoagulant found in tissue) and has anticoagulant properties.[4] Also remember that anything containing charcoal should be taken on an empty stomach to ensure that the charcoal doesn't absorb nutrients and minerals and reduce intestinal absorption of these nutrients. Do not take Potter's Acidosis at the same time as other medications. The charcoal can reduce your absorption of prescription medications.

References

[1] Farmakol Toksikol, 43(6):700-5, 1980

[2] Zhong Xi Yi Jie He Za Zhi, 10(3):150-1, 1990

[3] J Ethnopharmacol, 19(3):279-83, 1987

[4] Farmakol Toksikol, 53(4):39-41, 1990

CHAPTER 24

UriCare:
Herbal UTI and kidney stone treatment convinces even the biggest skeptics

Greta Kirby told us she was desperate. She had suffered from urinary tract infections off and on since she was a teenager. Using vitamin C therapy, she managed to avoid problems for a few years until early last summer. Then she got a new infection, a really bad one. She went to her doctor, who prescribed 14 days of Bactrim, a standard treatment for cases of severe, recurrent UTIs. But it didn't work, and she went back to her doctor, who put her on another antibiotic, Ampicillin, for 14 more days. Her symptoms began to lessen, but she was still experiencing discomfort and burning. "It was the worst hanger-on thing," she told us. "Whatever caused it, it was so strong that those antibiotics just couldn't get rid of all of it. And after taking all those prescriptions, I was at my wit's end."

We know that many of you can relate. Over the years, we've heard from numerous HSI readers struggling with recurrent infections who were frustrated with conventional treatments that proved to be ineffective, expensive, or riddled with side effects. Yet despite our continuing research, we hadn't heard of many simple, natural remedies for UTIs, so we were very interested in UriCare, a product made with ingredients from traditional Indian herbal medicine that gave Greta the relief she so dearly wanted.

Deciding to seek out an alternative treatment was a big step for Greta. "As a registered nurse, I must say all these herbal medicines are new to me, and I am the first to admit that I am pessimistic about them," she said. She confided that she has "some wacky friends that will take anything." (Hmmm, those "wacky friends" sound like some of us.)

Of course, a lot of us were skeptical about alternative medicine ourselves before we saw the benefits it could provide—and not all alternative therapies are valid. It seems every month we come across products and ingredients that don't do nearly what they claim they can.

Eliminate symptoms completely in just 48 hours

Certain parts of Greta's story gave us a definite feeling of déjà vu. She desperately wanted to feel better, so she researched a few products on the Internet before going to her favorite health food store where she got the recommendation for UriCare, a formula of Ayurvedic (traditional Indian medicinal) herbs used to treat urinary tract infections and kidney stones. Because she was determined to be "really, really careful," Greta called the company's medical director, Dr. Grace Ormstein, to discuss her condition

---

PASS KIDNEY STONES EASIER—AND PREVENT THEM FROM FORMING IN THE FIRST PLACE

It is an excruciating ordeal that has been described as more painful than childbirth. And every year, roughly one million Americans experience that terrible sensation of passing a kidney stone.

In the past few months, we've sent several e-Alerts on studies recommending dietary changes and herbal treatments for kidney stones (for information on how to sign up for free HSI e-Alerts see page 225). But we know that no one treatment will work for all of you, so we're always searching for additional alternatives you can try.

Kidney stones are recognized as one of the most common—and most painful—urinary tract disorders. A host of conditions contribute to their formation: kidney disorders, metabolic disorders (such as hyperparathyroidism), urinary tract infections, hereditary conditions, gout, diet, certain diuretics, calcium supplements, calcium-based antacids, and excessive intake of vitamin D. And, unfortunately, if you've had one kidney stone, you're likely to get another.

---

and the formula. Only then did she decide to give the supplement a try.

"It was unbelievable," Greta told us. "I took the first dose on a Friday afternoon. By Saturday night, I didn't have any more burning. I continued to take the product and after 48 hours, my symptoms had entirely vanished. It was the first relief I had had in a month."

So just what is UriCare? It's a formulation of seven botanicals (see sidebar on page 157) which has been used in India for the past 35 years. Like most other modern natural medicines, it has been tested in petri dishes and laboratory animals. Better still, it has been tested extensively in humans. While researching this story, we found 19 clinical trials involving a total of more

---

PASS KIDNEY STONES EASIER...*CONTINUED*

Researchers have attempted to produce a chemical agent capable of safely dissolving kidney stones within the body. And those efforts produced several pharmaceuticals. But at least one group of researchers was less than impressed with these so-called "wonder drugs." In a study we reviewed while preparing this article, the researchers said those drugs were good for nothing more than "washing the catheters and urinary containers."[1]

That's why several of the human trials of UriCare intrigued us: They demonstrated that UriCare can help people pass kidney stones and avoid developing subsequent stones—something pharmaceuticals just can't seem to do.

In one of these studies, researchers asked 255 individuals with kidney stones to take two capsules of UriCare twice a day. The subjects weren't given any other diuretics, anti-inflammatories, or anti-spasmodic drugs. An astounding 233 subjects (91.3 percent) expelled their stones within one to three months of beginning treatment. "Patients often returned with the expelled stone as a mark of gratitude to the prescribing doctor," the researchers noted. (We couldn't help thinking a thank-you note would

than 1,500 people—an impressive count for an alternative medicine. All the trials took place in India, and (surprise!) managed to escape the notice of American MDs, which probably explains why most of us had never heard of it before.

After reviewing the study results, we certainly can't say that UriCare is a wonder cure. The results were mixed. It didn't work for everyone. In fact, it didn't work for almost half the participants in one study. But those clinical trials documented hundreds of cases in which UriCare was able to ease and prevent two horribly uncomfortable conditions: urinary tract infections and kidney stones. In many cases, it provided faster relief, fewer side effects,

---

PASS KIDNEY STONES EASIER...*CONTINUED*

have done just fine.) And even better, of those 233 patients, 47 expelled the stone as sand-like material, suggesting the UriCare can actually dissolve the stone within the body. Only 22 of the patients had stones that had to be removed mechanically.[2]

UriCare proves four times more effective than prescription drugs

Another study involving 100 people compared the ability of UriCare and a prescription antispasmodic to induce the passage of kidney stones. The UriCare proved nearly four times more effective, enabling 39 people to pass their stones, as opposed to just 11 of the people taking the antispasmodic drug.[3]

When we talked to Dr. Ormstein, she told me she talked with numerous people who have used UriCare to treat their kidney stones. She says the stones typically pass within two to three weeks. And many times, they come out as sand, which dramatically reduces the amount of pain caused by their elimination.

and cheaper treatment than leading pharmaceuticals. In some cases, it augmented the effect of those drugs.

Traditional herbal blend offers UTI cure where conventional medicine falls short

Urinary tract infections account for more than eight million doctor visits in the United States alone each year. More than 20 percent of American women will get a UTI at some point in their lives, and many of those women will get multiple UTIs. (If you're female and you've already had three urinary tract infections, chances are, you are going to keep getting more.)

A number of conditions can make you susceptible to a UTI: any abnormality

---

PASS KIDNEY STONES EASIER...*CONTINUED*

A few studies suggest that UriCare may help prevent new stones from forming. Researchers haven't yet done any long-term studies to track recurrence rates among kidney stone patients who take UriCare. Rather, their assumption comes from urine analyses done on people who repeatedly develop kidney stones. Those analyses show that treatment with UriCare changes the chemical composition of urine. Specifically, it lowers levels of calcium and oxalic acid (two substances known to contribute to the formation of kidney stones) and raises levels of phosphorus (a substance known to inhibit the creation of kidney stones). So it would make sense that the individuals are less likely to develop new stones. For ordering information see the Source Directory starting on page 213.

As we said in the beginning of this chapter, results on UriCare have been mixed. If you decide to give it a try, please write in or go to the website forum at www.hsibaltimore.com and let us know whether it worked for you.

---

that obstructs urine flow (such as a kidney stone), diabetes, an enlarged prostate, or having to use a catheter. But the reality is that some people are just susceptible.

The symptoms range from uncomfortable to highly painful: a frequent (and sometimes urgent) need to urinate; a burning feeling in the bladder; and sometimes an overall feeling of being tired, shaky and washed out.

"Prolonged conditions, especially chronic urinary tract infections, tend to cause a lot of scarring in the urethra," Dr. Grace Ormstein told us. "This makes things worse because it causes spasms and makes it very painful for the urethra to release urine." Some women even have to undergo surgery to correct the condition and relieve the pain. Untreated UTIs have been known to cause kidney failure, an overload of toxins in the bloodstream, dementia-like symptoms, and even death.

The conventional treatment is antibiotics. Unfortunately, they can't always clear severe infections, they don't always prevent recurrences, and women who suffer from chronic UTIs often become drug-resistant.

UriCare, however, has demonstrated an ability to both treat and prevent urinary tract infections. In small studies, its track record of relieving UTIs has varied. In one study, it cured 100 percent of cases.[4] In another, it provided "good to excellent" relief from symptoms for 51 percent of participants.[5] While those results are promising, I want to point out that they're not evidence of a sure-fire cure.

Cut UTI healing time in half and reduce the cost of your treatment by 25 percent

One large-scale trial, however, did produce compelling evidence that a combination of Indian herbs and modern pharmaceuticals could provide highly effective therapy for UTIs. It compared the ability of UriCare and pharmaceuticals to treat and prevent UTIs in 297 people over the course of two years.[6]

The first phase of the study assessed the ability of different medications to cure acute UTIs. Patients who received pharmaceutical treatment (an

(continued on page 158)

ONCE AGAIN, LOOKING TO THE PAST UNLOCKS A HEALTHIER FUTURE

Ayurveda (which translates from Sanskrit as "knowledge of life") is probably the world's oldest system of natural medicine, dating back more than 6,000 years ago.

In 1930, the Himalaya Drug Company of Bangalore, India began formulating herbal remedies, based on Ayurvedic knowledge, and subjecting them to modern, pharmaceutical testing. Himalaya's researchers combined seven botanicals in UriCare (also known as Cystone). They are:

- **Shilapushpa** – The leaves of this small herb have been used in Ayurvedic medicine to treat kidney and bladder stones by causing their disintegration and expulsion. The leaves also produce a number of antifungal compounds.

- **Pasanabheda** – According to Ayurvedic teachings, the root of this perennial herb acts as a diuretic, laxative, astringent and anti-infective agent. It helps dissolve kidney gravel and stones by correcting the balance of colloids (a gelatinous substance) and crystalloids in the kidneys.

- **Rough Chaff Tree** (Achyranthes aspera) – The seeds from this spikey herb are reported to be a strong astringent and diuretic.

- **Indian Madder** (Rubia cordifolia) – The roots of this prickly creeper contain an acid that has proven to dissolve stones in the urinary tract.

- **Ash Colored Fleabane** (Vernonia cinerea) – A plant reported to be useful in controlling bladder spasms.

- **Umbrella's Edge** (Cyerus scariosus) and **Sedge** (Onosma bracteatum) – Two diuretics.

alkalizer and an antimicrobial), were cured in an average of 9 to 12 days. Patients who received UriCare along with the pharmaceuticals (some received UriCare plus both drugs, some received just UriCare and an alkalizer) were cured in 6 days. In addition to healing faster, the UriCare + alkalizer patients suffered absolutely no side effects. Patients receiving other treatments experienced occasional indigestion, diarrhea and flatulence. Furthermore, the UriCare patients knocked down the cost of their treatment by 25 percent. (And given the present state of drug prices, HMO premiums, and Medicare legislation, a 25 percent savings can really add up.)

The second phase of the study assessed the ability of different treatments to prevent recurrences of UTIs. Patients received either an ongoing maintenance dose of an antimicrobial, daily doses of UriCare alone, or daily doses of UriCare and the antimicrobial. The researchers concluded that UriCare alone was the superior treatment. Only five people suffered a recurrence in two years and just seven experienced any side effects (specifically, indigestion and flatulence). Among the people receiving drug treatment, 16 suffered a recurrence and everyone experienced side effects. (The combination treatment produced mixed results: just two people had recurrences but everyone struggled with side effects.) UriCare carried the added benefit of being the cheaper maintenance therapy.

We asked Greta if she took UriCare throughout the year. She said no, but that she has taken the supplement for a few days whenever she has felt another UTI coming on and has successfully avoided flare-ups. Consequently a year later, she's still UTI-free—and has a nearly full bottle of UriCare sitting on her shelf!

For information on ordering UriCare see the Source Directory starting on page 213.

References

[1] Medicine and Surgery, December 21, 1993

[2] Medicine and Surgery, December 21, 1993

[3] Curr Med Pract, 5:26, 1982

[4] Probe, 1:27, 1982

[5] Probe, 4:270, 1980

[6] Curr Med Pract, (35) 4: 89, 1991

Conquering Diabetes

There is no known cure for diabetes. And there may never be. But if you have diabetes you **can** live a long healthy life managing—and in some cases even eliminating—the symptoms.

We are literally facing an epidemic of diabetes today, with over a million new cases being diagnosed a year. With 17 million diabetics in the United States alone there are few of us that have not been somehow touched by this disease. Whether you have received the devastating diagnosis, been given a warning by your doctor that you have risk factors for diabetes, or watched a loved one suffer with this disease the following section should be of interest to you.

In this next section you will learn about six highly promising herbal diabetes-fighters that come straight from the Amazon. You will read about a variety of approaches for controlling blood sugar levels and get tips on techniques that could slash your risk of developing diabetes in half! And you will discover a truly novel approach to smashing your sugar addiction that might help you *kick the habit* once and for all.

Glucotor:
Dodge the sugar bullet–and double your chances of beating this leading killer

There's an unfolding epidemic of what folks were still calling "sugar diabetes" when many of us were growing up. Over the last decade, the number of Americans diagnosed with diabetes increased by 50 percent. Today, 17 million Americans have diabetes—and the number will top 22 million by 2005.[1]

Over the same time frame, there was a major jump in obesity rates, too, up 57 percent. Of course, it isn't just sugar that makes a body fat, but it helps—especially when the average American eats 152 pounds of it each year. We know it's hard to believe, especially if you don't eat sweets or drink sugared soft drinks. But some of that sugar is in processed and preserved foods in the form of sucrose, corn syrup, caramel color, or fructose. And some of it's in pasta and other refined carbohydrates that turn into sugar when they reach our digestive systems.

The sad fact is that simply following a "normal" American diet can put us at risk of developing type 2 diabetes. Also known as adult-onset diabetes, this type of the disease accounts for up to 95 percent of all cases and is the kind ballooning to epidemic proportions.

The cost of mainstream diabetes treatment: $10,000 a year <u>and</u> your health

You're at greater risk for type 2 if a family member has the condition. But lifestyle choices, including diet, can trigger or prevent it. Too much sugar can stress and potentially damage your body's ability to produce and absorb insulin.

Diabetes is a difficult disease to manage. The average diabetic requires over $10,000 in medical products and services annually. Even with good medical management, diabetics are at increased risk of heart disease, stroke, blindness, kidney failure, and limb amputations. Every year, more than 200,000 Americans die from diabetes-related complications.

Treatment for type 2 diabetes often includes oral medications. Yet at least one of them proved to be as dangerous as the disease. Over 400 deaths were linked to Rezulin, which was prescribed to 750,000 Americans between 1997 and 2000, when it was withdrawn from the market. Some patient advocates believe that the number of deaths may have been 10 times as many—and that's not including future deaths due to cirrhosis caused or hastened by the drug.[2]

At the time it took Rezulin off the market, the Food and Drug Administration (FDA) steered patients to two newer drugs, Avandia and Actos, in the same category. Both were recommended as offering the same benefits as Rezulin but with lower risks.[3] They're still on the market today, with a warning (among others) to watch for signs of liver disease and check liver enzymes regularly. When we checked the National Diabetes Information Clearinghouse, it listed these along with 17 other brands of diabetes pills (complete with their generic names) for a total of 19 pills and seven types of medicine.[4] Need we add that each comes listed with side effects ranging from unpleasant (a metallic taste in the mouth) to downright scary (liver failure, kidney damage)?

Always on the lookout for alternative approaches to treating type 2 diabetes, we talked recently with a couple of our HSI panelists. Leslie Taylor told us about the product she's developed and made available to patients through physicians. It's a tea that includes several botanicals from the Amazon—including pata de vaca, pedra hume caa, bitter melon and chanca piedra—all of which have demonstrated an ability to lower blood sugar levels. And Jon Barron gave us a detailed explanation of his work in developing a natural diabetes formula.

Change of heart leads to sugar-busting breakthrough

For years, Jon had resisted suggestions that he devise an approach for battling diabetes. His reluctance, he told us, stemmed from his belief that using formulas to manage the symptoms of diabetes without dealing with the underlying causes ultimately fails. The responsible approach, he thought, was to help people optimize the health of the organs in the body that control blood sugar levels—not to treat the symptoms after people had the disease.

But the realities of the American diet finally changed his mind, and he began to look at botanicals that could actually accomplish both things simultaneously, help control blood sugar levels and help rebuild the organs that control those levels—not just in diabetics and pre-diabetics, but in anyone eating a less than perfect diet.

Doing our own research, we have come across a number of herbs, including milk thistle, bitter melon, ginseng, and aloe, used to control blood sugar. Ayurvedic medicine offers more than 44 different herbal therapies and formulas for diabetes. Both fenugreek and gymnema, for example, come from this tradition. And in our searches, we found that these two have been the subject of 30 different studies of varying degrees of scientific rigor in Indian and Western literature. Only two did not favor the treatment being tested.

This potent pair of sugar controllers shown effective in 93 percent of studies

After investigating a number of botanicals, Jon Barron settled on four. The first two come from the Ayurvedic tradition and the third from Japan. We found extensive research, including clinical trials, on these three. The fourth, nopal cactus, has a folk tradition in the American Southwest and Mexico; research on it is promising, but not as extensive as the others.

It's worth noting that several of these botanicals also impact high blood pressure and abnormal blood lipid levels, both characteristics of pre-diabetes, as well as blood sugar levels. Evidence suggests that one even regenerates cells in the pancreas, which, in turn, facilitates healthier insulin levels.

Blood sugar levels plummet by 30 percent with one herb

Seeds from fenugreek plants (*Trigonella foenum-gracum*) have long been used in India, Africa, and the Middle East to treat gastrointestinal problems, gout, wounds, hyperlipidemia, and diabetes. Clinical research dating back to 1939 suggests that fenugreek helps normalize how the body absorbs and uses glucose. The seeds contain a rare type of fiber that forms a gel inside the stomach, reducing its ability to absorb sugar and fat. The gel also makes the stomach feel full faster and longer, promoting weight loss.

On average, participants in fenugreek clinical trials have seen their fasting blood sugar drop by 30 percent, their sugar levels after eating drop 20-35 percent, and their hemoglobin A1C drop by 12 percent. (The A1C test is an index of diabetes severity that measures the average amount of sugar molecules that have attached to red blood cells.) In one study, participants experienced a 54 percent drop in urinary glucose levels.[5]

Other clinical trials have shown that fenugreek can reduce total cholesterol, LDL and triglyceride levels, particularly in individuals suffering from coronary artery disease and type 2 diabetes.[6,7] In short, it may help diabetics reduce both their blood sugar and blood lipid levels.

However, the news isn't all good. To get those effects, some study participants had to take large amounts—as much as 100 grams a day—of a herb that tastes acutely bitter and makes for foul smelling sweat and urine. In addition, fenugreek can trigger some side effects, specifically cramping, diarrhea, flatulence and other gastrointestinal disorders. But a recently developed extract eliminates some side effects (specifically, the taste and odor) and concentrates the active ingredient, making smaller doses possible. Fenugreek, however, is still contraindicated in some circumstances. Because of its high fiber content, it can alter your absorption of other medications (such as

(continued on page 166)

FIVE THINGS YOU CAN DO TODAY TO SLASH YOUR RISK IN HALF

This year, a million new cases of diabetes will be diagnosed. Another 5.9 million Americans who have the disease still won't know that they do.[8] In addition, over 30 percent of Americans are "pre-diabetic" and stand to develop full-blown diabetes in five to 10 years.

So how do you avoid becoming one of the millions who will be diagnosed with this disease? It's actually quite simple: understand and reduce your risk.[9]

FIVE THINGS YOU CAN DO TODAY...*CONTINUED*

Some risks you can't help:

- Being over 45 years old
- Having a parent or sibling with diabetes
- Being African American, Hispanic American, Asian American, American Indian, or Pacific Islander
- And, for women only, developing diabetes during pregnancy (gestational diabetes) or giving birth to a baby nine pounds or bigger.

But other risk factors are within your control:

- Excess weight (more than 80 percent of people with type 2 diabetes are overweight)
- High blood pressure (especially if it is 140/90 or higher)
- Abnormal cholesterol levels (an HDL cholesterol level of 35 or lower, triglyceride levels of 250 or higher)
- An inactive lifestyle (e.g., you exercise less than three times a week)
- Excess dietary sugars and carbohydrates.

If you're over 45 and have any other risk factor, you should get a blood glucose test at least once every three years. In addition to diagnosing diabetes, the test can identify "pre-diabetes"—a condition with blood sugar readings that are above normal but below diabetic level. High blood pressure and abnormal cholesterol levels often accompany these elevated blood sugars.

Learning that you're pre-diabetic can give you a chance to delay or entirely prevent the onset of diabetes by making a few lifestyle changes.

Recent research indicates that a healthy diet and moderate, regular exercise can cut a person's risk of developing diabetes by 58 percent.

anticoagulants, MAO inhibitors, and hypoglycemic medications) and change their effectiveness.

Herbal "sugar killer" makes sweets hit a sour note

A woody vine used in Indian medicine for over 2,000 years, gymnema sylvestre is commonly known as the "sugar destroyer." A peptide found in the plant blocks certain receptor sites on our taste buds and eventually makes sugar taste, well, not sweet.[10] But gymnema does more to ease diabetes symptoms than quell our sugar cravings.

Gymnemic acid (a key active ingredient) fills sugar receptor sites in the intestine, too, making them unavailable to ingested sugars. If the sugar you eat doesn't get digested, it doesn't filter into your bloodstream. Clinical research also indicates that gymnema regenerates beta cells in the pancreas (which are involved in insulin production), stimulates the release of increased amounts of insulin, and increases the permeability of cells so that they absorb more insulin.[11]

Several clinical studies have measured gymnema's effect on both type 1 and type 2 diabetes. Type 1 diabetics who took 400 mg for 6 to 30 months saw their blood sugar levels drop 52.6 percent on average.[12] Most participants in an 18-month study achieved such significant and consistent blood sugar decreases that they were able to reduce their medication. Five participants were able to discontinue insulin use entirely and maintain healthy blood sugar levels by taking only 400 mg of gymnema sylvestre extract daily.[13]

To date, no one has reported experiencing adverse side effects from the herb, and it is not contraindicated for any condition. No tests, however, have been conducted to determine whether it can be safely taken by pregnant women.

Ancient blood sugar controlling secret also drops blood pressure and cholesterol

You've probably never heard of konjac mannan (we sure hadn't before we started researching this article), but it's been used as a food remedy for over 1,000 years in Japan. And it's also been tested in a number of clinical trials. In a 65-day trial, 72 patients with adult-onset diabetes who took konjac saw their fasting blood sugar levels drop an average of 51.8 percent and their levels after eating drop 84.6 percent.[14] In an eight-week trial, pre-diabetics reported improvements in their blood sugar and cholesterol levels. On average, their total cholesterol dropped by 12.4 percent, LDL levels dropped by 22 percent, and LDL/HDL ratios fell by 22.2 percent.[15]

Other benefits have been reported for konjac. Patients with type 2 diabetes also suffering from high cholesterol and high blood pressure experienced an average drop in their systolic blood pressure of 6.9 percent after supplementing with konjac mannan.[16] Twenty obese individuals who took konjac for eight weeks lost an average of 5.5 pounds even though they were explicitly told not to change their diet or exercise routines. They also experienced significant reductions in their LDL and total cholesterol levels.[17]

At the University of Toronto, researchers concluded that konjac mannan extract is two to four times more effective than pectin, psyllium, guar, oats, and other fibers at reducing cholesterol. It also proved to be equally effective as statin drugs at lowering LDL cholesterol and as some conventional diabetic agents, such as Acarbose, at controlling blood sugar levels.[18]

Fiber-rich Indian remedy solves prickly problem of sugar/fat conversion

Leaves from the nopal cactus, commonly known as the prickly pear cactus, have long been regarded as health food by native peoples in Mexico and southwestern United States. There's not a lot of clinical research into the botanical's medicinal benefits, but anecdotal evidence and several small studies suggest that eating nopal leaves with a meal can help contain and even reduce serum glucose levels.[19] Individuals with type 2 diabetes have experienced a 10 to 20 percent reduction in blood sugar levels after eating nopal. Researchers aren't certain how nopal lowers blood sugar, but they suggest that its rich fiber content inhibits the absorption of glucose in the intestinal tract.

A larger body of research indicates that nopal can reduce both cholesterol and triglyceride levels.[20] Researchers have suggested that it accomplishes this by eliminating excess bile acids (which eventually turn into cholesterol) and by inhibiting the conversion of blood sugar into fat.

This four-in-one solution kicks sugar and fat metabolism into overdrive

These four botanicals make up what Jon Barron refers to as his "sugar, lipid metabolic enhancement formula," officially called Glucotor. It's designed to offset the impact of high-sugar, high-fat foods. In pre-diabetics and non-diabetics, it can help promote healthier blood sugar and cholesterol levels...and a healthier weight. Jon told us he takes it himself on occasion and avoids the sleepiness that follows a few hours after indulging in a meal that's a little too rich or too sweet.

For diabetics, Glucotor may have even bigger ramifications. Although the formula hasn't undergone clinical trials, one physician has tested it in his family practice in Evansville, Indiana on diabetic patients. According to Barron, "It produced results that the doctors have not seen before, even with hard core drugs," including dramatic changes in blood sugar levels.

Patients find fast diabetes and hypertension relief—without prescription drugs

To find out more, we called Anthony Hall, M.D., the physician in Indiana. It turns out that he's in training to be a naturopathic doctor, and he was happy to provide information on the 15 patients who agreed to take the formula.

Three of them, he told us, dropped out of the trial due to digestive problems caused by the product. (The formula can stimulate large, urgent bowel movements, so people just starting the supplement may want to take only half of the standard daily dose and give their digestive systems a chance to adjust.)

He monitored the effect of Glucotor on his patients' blood sugar, blood pressure, and cholesterol levels, and cautions that, if you're on medication to control any of those levels, you absolutely should consult with your doctor before trying Glucotor and arrange to have your levels checked regularly.

One of Dr. Hall's patients was a 56-year-old woman who had been on varying doses of insulin and oral hypoglycemics since she was diagnosed with diabetes in 1993. Before she began taking Glucotor, her hemoglobin A1C level was 9.0. (A reading of 9 indicates severe diabetes, while 6 or less indicates a healthy, non-diabetic condition.) Over the course of taking Glucotor for six weeks, she discontinued her insulin and Metformin (the generic form of Glucophage, one of the most common prescription drugs used to treat diabetes) and reduced her oral hypoglycemic from 8 mg to 2 mg per day. At the end of the trial, a second test showed her A1C level had fallen to 5.7, a healthy, non-diabetic level.

During our conversation, Dr. Hall also told us how surprised he was to see dramatic changes in blood lipid levels in some of his Glucotor patients. One man's total cholesterol dropped from 297 to 210 and his triglycerides from 580 to 506 after four weeks of taking the supplement. Another patient, a woman this time, had a 23.5 percent reduction in her total cholesterol, a 32 percent drop in her LDL level, and an 18 percent drop in her triglycerides. After 5.5 weeks of taking Glucotor, her blood pressure dropped from 140/96 to around 115/75, and she was able to discontinue taking Lipitor and her blood pressure medication.

And these are just a few examples of the great responses Dr. Hall saw in his patients. Of course, Glucotor isn't for everyone. The side effects that caused the three patients to drop out of Dr. Hall's study may be more than you anticipated or are willing to encounter. But the main point here is that type 2 diabetes isn't just an epidemic that is coming and none of us can avoid. There are plenty of steps you can take to head it off at the pass in your own life. If enough of us do, maybe we can make type 2 diabetes into "the epidemic that wasn't." It's certainly worth a try.

For information on ordering Glucotor see the Source Directory starting on page 213.

References

1. Centers for Disease Control

2. "Over 400 Fatalities Made Rezulin A Deadly Diabetes Medicine," Herman, Mathis, Kasey, Kitchens, & Gerel, LLP (www.hermanmathis-rezulin.com)

3. "Diabetes drug Rezulin taken off market." CNN (www.cnn.com), 3/22/00

4. National institute of Diabetes & Digestive & Kidney Diseases website (www.niddk.nih.gov)

5. Eur J Clin Nutr 1990; 44(4): 301-6

6. Prostaglandins Leukot Essent Fatty Acids 1997; 56 (5): 379-384

7. Plant Foods Hum Nutr 1999; 53(4): 359-365

8. Centers for Disease Control

9. National Institutes of Health

10. J Biochem (Tokyo) 1992; 111(1): 109-112

11. J. Endocrinol 1999; 163 (2): 207-212

12. J Ethnopharmacol 1990; 30: 281-294

13. J. Ethnopharmacol 1990; 30(3): 295-300

14. Bio Environ Sci 1990 Jun; 3(2): 123-131

15. Diabetes Care 2000; 23(1): 9-14

16. Diabetes Care 1999; 22(6): 913-919

17. Int J Obes 1984; 8(4): 289-293

18. Diabetes Care 1999; 22(6): 1-7

19. "Medical Implications of Prickly Pear Cactus," Texas A&M University (www.tamuk.edu)

20. Gac Med Mex 1992; 128(4): 431-436

Pancreas Support:
Six diabetes-fighting secrets straight from the Amazon

You've heard this before, but it bears repeating: We're living in the midst of a diabetes epidemic. Diagnoses have increased by 50 percent over the last decade in the U.S., and people over age 65 make up more than 20 percent of that population.

In the last chapter we wrote about an herbal sugar control remedy called glucotor, brought to our attention by HSI panelist Jon Barron. (See page 223 for information on becoming a member of the Health Sciences Institute). Glucotor is a blend of four ancient herbs that have been clinically proven to reduce blood sugar levels and improve sugar and fat metabolism.

But there's more. Just recently, HSI panelist Leslie Taylor told us about a new natural remedy for blood sugar control. We think you'll be impressed— its ingredients are so powerful, many of them have been referred to as "vegetable insulins." They're heavily relied upon in the Amazon, where diabetes is just as prevalent as it is here and where most don't have access to pharmaceutical drugs...much less to electricity to run a refrigerator to store insulin. So, as you can see, there's good reason why they've developed—and rely upon—herbal alternatives.

Mother Nature gives you direct control over your blood sugar and insulin levels

This herbal formula is a blend of six substances, some of which will be familiar to long-time HSI members. *Pata de vaca, pedra hume caa, bitter melon, chanca piedra,* and *stevia* are all derived from native South American plants, and have been used for centuries in that continent's traditional healing practices. (You may also be familiar with chanca piedra as a kidney stone therapy [see the sidebar on page 172], and stevia as a sweetener.) The sixth is *neem*, a leading antidiabetic and pancreas supportive herb from India.

The first five herbs have a long history of use in South America and the Amazon for abnormal blood sugar levels. Pata de vaca (Latin name *Bauhinia forficata*) has been used to balance blood sugar levels for over 60 years, and is also used to treat complications of diabetes like kidney disorders, polyuria (large urine volume), and other urinary problems. In a 2002 Brazilian study, researchers found that diabetic rats treated with pata de vaca showed "a significant reduction in serum and urinary glucose and urinary urea" as compared to controls.[1]

Pedra hume caa (Latin name *Myrcia uniflora*) was first dubbed "vegetable

---

CHANCA PIEDRA: THE NATURAL "STONE BREAKER"

The Amazon herb chanca piedra is one ingredient in the blood sugar control herbal blend Pancreas Support. But it is probably better known for its ability to effectively break up and prevent kidney stones, an agonizing condition that affects 5 1/2 million people in the U.S. alone.

Chanca piedra has been proven to not only ease the passing of kidney stones but also help prevent them from forming in the first place. In our research, we found that it was 94 percent successful in eliminating stones. And in a 1999 study, researchers confirmed that chanca piedra has a "**potent and effective**" inhibitory effect on the formation of calcium-oxalate crystals (the building blocks of most kidney stones).

If you've suffered through the pain of kidney stones, chances are you'd be willing to try just about anything to avoid going through it again. That's why we were so excited when we discovered chanca piedra. We first told our members about this natural herb from the Amazon rain forest in the September 2000 issue of the HSI Members Alert newsletter. Since then, countless readers have written, called, and e-mailed to thank us for it. See the Source Directory starting on page 213 to learn how you can order.

---

insulin" in 1965 by noted Brazilian herbalist Dr. C.L. Cruz, and its efficacy has been supported by clinical research. In one 1990 study, scientists performed a randomized crossover double-blind study of pedra hume caa with a group of healthy subjects and a group of diabetic subjects. They found that the herb effectively lowered plasma insulin levels in the diabetic subjects.[2]

Bitter melon (Latin name *Momordica charantia*) is both a food and a medicine in the Amazon. The fruit is traditionally used to treat diabetes, as well as infections, hepatitis, parasites, and other ailments. In a 2002 Indian study, scientists found that bitter melon significantly reduced plasma glucose levels in diabetic rats in as little as one month and that the effects continually increased over a period of four months.[3]

In Brazilian herbal medicine, chanca piedra is called *quebra pedra* and has been used to treat a wide variety of health issues. While chanca piedra is best known for its effectiveness against kidney stones, as we first reported in the September 2000 issue of the HSI *Members Alert*, Brazilian traditional medicine has also relied upon the herb to help regulate blood sugar. These effects were validated in a 1995 Indian study that found that chanca piedra (Latin name *Phyllanthus niruri*) "**significantly reduced**" blood glucose levels in people with diabetes.[4]

That brings us to stevia. We find it interesting that a formula designed to control blood sugar contains this natural sweetener, which is known to be 300 times sweeter than cane sugar. Yet despite its intense flavor, stevia does not raise blood sugar levels—in fact, it can help lower them. One recent study showed that stevia suppressed glucose response and increased insulin response in diabetic rats.[5]

As we said, the sixth ingredient in this special formula is neem (Latin name *Azadirachta indica*)—an herb from Indian medicine. A 1999 study of four plants known to lower blood sugar found neem the most potent, and animal studies have documented the herb's effectiveness in controlling sugar in both normal and diabetic rabbits.[6-8] In 2000, researchers concluded that "[neem] could be of benefit in diabetes mellitus in controlling the blood sugar or may also be helpful in preventing or delaying the onset of the disease."

Unique blend offers another weapon in the war against diabetes

As you can see, centuries of tradition and dozens of modern research studies show that each of these individual ingredients can help control blood sugar. So Leslie Taylor was intrigued to find out what all of them could do together. And that's just what Raintree Nutrition has done, blending the dried leaves of pata de vaca, pedra hume caa, bitter melon, chanca piedra, stevia, and neem into one complete formulation. Raintree calls the blend Pancreas Support; the recommended usage is two to three capsules with each meal. For ordering information please see the Source Directory starting on page 213.

Only you can decide what's best for you, but Pancreas Support offers you another choice for safe, natural blood sugar balancing and another way to help maintain your good health.

References

[1] (1) J Ethnopharmacol 2002; 81: 191-197

[2] Braz J Med Biol Res 1990; 23: 11-20

[3] Phytother Res 2002; 16: 236-243

[4] Indian J Exp Biol 1995; 33: 861-864

[5] Phytomedicine 2002; 9: 9-14

[6] Ethnopharmacol 1999; 67: 377-372

[7] Indian J Exp Biol 1992; 30: 1,170-1,175

[8] Gen Pharmacol 1996; 27: 431-434

Sugar Blocker:
Forget willpower: Overcome sugar addiction in 21 days with a natural herb

If it's ever happened to you, you know it's something far beyond willpower. Maybe you're driving home from work, maybe you're reading a gripping murder mystery. But all of a sudden your thoughts turn to a leftover piece of cake in the fridge. You're not even hungry and you know you don't need the extra calories, but you literally cannot stop thinking about it. Finally, you get to the fridge, fork in hand, and you give in. It isn't a lack of willpower that got you, it's a full-fledged addiction.

The same brain receptors that can lead to drug and nicotine addictions also let you become addicted to sugar.[1]

Understanding that it's *not* personal weakness, but a true physical addiction, is the first step to overcoming the cravings. Let's be honest: It's not easy to give up sugar. Cravings—physical and mental—can dominate your thoughts. Quitting "cold turkey" sometimes works to curb cravings, but that can backfire. Avoiding sweets can lead to such an uncontrollable craving for sugar that you "give in" just once—and end up bingeing. And then the cycle continues.

Pavlov's dogs hold one key to beating your habit

Research shows that certain activities or habits (like sitting down to that mystery novel) may be compelling you to eat sugary foods. This goes back to the studies done by Pavlov. We all remember the story of how he conditioned dogs to salivate when a bell rang by ringing a bell whenever they were fed. Eventually, the dogs began to salivate just from the sound of the bell—food was no longer required.

Your sugar habit may have a similar psychological connection. You may crave sugar because of certain surroundings, smells, sounds, or circumstances.[2] If, for example, you always eat a candy bar when you go to the movies, then viewing a film on your VCR may stimulate the same cravings. This sort of behavior pattern becomes an even bigger problem when the frequency of the activity increases: You probably watch movies at home more often than you do at the theater. If you give in to your sugar cravings each time you pop a video into the VCR, you'll significantly increase your sugar intake.

"Just for the taste of it" puts you back at the beginning

For some people, changing their behavior is all that's needed to stop eating sugar. But, if you crave sugar because you're dependent on it or are physically addicted to it, environmental and behavioral changes probably won't halt the incessant cravings. And it's important to note that switching over to artificial sweeteners won't help.

It's the sweet *taste* that generates the release of addiction-building brain chemicals. According to Dr. Bart Hoebel, a neuroscience addiction researcher at Princeton University, the surge of dopamine and opioids—brain chemicals that "drive" the addiction process—occurs regardless of the number of calories in the sweetening agent.[3]

Dr. Hoebel's animal research indicates that rats experiencing sugar withdrawal displayed symptoms such as teeth-chattering, anxiety, and "high-pitched crying." These are classic displays of withdrawal from an addictive substance, although Dr. Hoebel claimed they were milder than those suffering from drug withdrawal.

If your sugar cravings are linked to dependence or addiction, you should expect to go through some withdrawal if you don't eat or drink something sweet when your body signals a need. Again, the symptoms of sugar withdrawal are similar to those of drug withdrawal, though not as severe.

Don't "tell" your brain that you're eating sugar

To break the endless cycle of sugar cravings, you have to address your <u>physical</u> requirement for a "hit" of something sweet as well as the <u>behavior</u> that automatically makes you reach for something sweet—even if you don't crave it at that moment.

There are different taste buds on your tongue. In order for you to taste something, it must touch the appropriate taste receptor, or bud, on your tongue. When the taste bud receives its "signal," it sends an impulse to the brain—and you know what flavor you're eating. If you eat something sweet but your tongue doesn't perceive it, it won't send the appropriate signal to your brain.[4]

Gymnema sylvestre, an herb well known by diabetics for reducing high blood-sugar levels, can prevent you from tasting sugar. When gymnema comes in contact with the taste buds on your tongue, it "binds" with the ones that receive the signal for sweet flavors and blocks the taste of sweet things from being perceived by your tongue.[5] Since your tongue doesn't know it's eating something sweet, it won't signal your brain's receptors to release opioids and dopamine.

Although the brain secretions of opioids and dopamine have been prevented, the chemistry of your brain has not been altered.[6] But it *does* mean you're defeating the cycle of physical addiction by stopping sweet flavors from "communicating" with your taste buds. It also means your brain's addiction receptors are not receiving a sugar fix. This may send you into some form of withdrawal.

Chew your way beyond the craving

Gymnema is available in capsule form at most health food stores, but it's inconvenient and messy to open a pill and pour the herb on your tongue whenever you want to avoid sweets. (Not to mention the look you'd get at the Dairy Queen.) Many people also find that gymnema has an unpleasant flavor. The ideal solution is to find a way to put gymnema on your tongue without all these hassles.

That's exactly what the research team at American BioSciences has done. They've developed a product called Sugar Blocker that combines gymnema with a gum base. By chewing on one or two pieces of the gum for 10-15 minutes, you can stop your taste buds from tasting sweet flavors.

Of course, not tasting sweets is only part of the solution for sugar cravings. If you don't stop the cravings from happening in the first place, you'll find yourself chewing gum all day long and still not get relief from the constant cravings.

In order to break your sugar cravings, you need to retrain yourself. Otherwise, the cravings will continue, and you run the risk of going on a sugar binge if you give in to those nagging urges.

Break the cycle for good—in less than a month

To properly retrain your brain, the researchers at American BioSciences suggest the following plan:

At the first sign of a sugar craving, chew one or two pieces of Sugar Blocker gum. After 10-15 minutes, you'll no longer be able to taste the sweet flavor of the gum. This is a sign that your tongue's receptors have been bound and can no longer taste sweets.

Eat whatever food you were craving before you chewed the gum. This step is essential because it will "teach" you to not crave that food. Since you can't taste sugar, you'll only taste the other flavors in the food or beverage. Cookies may taste like salty boards. Both sugar and milk sugar (lactose) will

---

EATING SWEETS FUELS CANCER GROWTH

One of the most devastating side effects of sugar consumption is accelerated cancer growth. Seventy years ago, Otto Warburg, Ph.D., won the Nobel Prize in medicine when he discovered that cancer cells use glucose (sugar) for growth. All cells have a requirement for glucose, but cancer cells have a much greater need. In fact, they're unable to multiply rapidly without it.

Besides fueling cancer growth, other health problems may be linked to eating too much sugar. In addition to causing obesity, excess sugar intake can lead to diabetes, encourage an overgrowth of pathogenic intestinal flora, aggravate gout, and cause or exacerbate panic attacks, hyperactivity, and depression. Not to mention what it does to your teeth!

---

be blocked in ice cream. Alcohol will be affected since it's also a form of sugar. Cake, fruit, candy, gum—anything that has a sweet taste will no longer send a sugar signal to your brain.

When you start to eat the foods you crave, you'll notice that your craving will disappear because the object of your craving tastes different than what you thought it would. (Fulfillment of your expectations is one of the reinforcing agents in the sugar cycle.) If things taste different than what you thought, then you may not crave it anymore. The purpose of the retraining process is to give you a new habit—one that doesn't crave sweets. Since sweets won't taste very good, you won't want to respond to your cravings. And your brain will stop releasing substances that drive you to eat more sweets.

Get "first dibs" before everyone jumps on this limited quantity band wagon

Obviously there are numerous health problems that can come from a sugar addiction—obesity, diabetes, anxiety, depression, and more. If you eat or drink a lot of sweets and suffer from these or other medical problems, you may be able to help clear them up or reduce their grip by breaking your addiction to sweets. (If you're diabetic, you should discuss your use of Sugar Blocker with your physician. It could actually reduce your insulin requirements.)

Sugar Blocker is available from American Bio-Sciences through Harmony Company. Just recently introduced to the market, Sugar Blocker is available in very limited quantities. For additional ordering information see the Source Directory starting on page 213.

References
[1] Rat studies show evidence of "sugar dependence." Reuters Health News, June 18, 2001
[2] Trends in Neurosciences, 24(8): 443, 2001
[3] Eur J Biochem, 264(2):525-33, 1999
[4] Am J Physiol Regul Intergr Comp Physiol, 278(6):R1513-7, 2000
[5] Eur J Biochem, 264(2):525-33, 1999
[6] Eur J Biochem, 264(2):525-33, 1999

Heart Healthy Solutions

As we age statistics tell us our chance of developing a heart-related disease rises. In fact around 40% of the approximate 25,100,000 Americans currently diagnosed with a heart related disease are age 65 or over. As our population ages that number is expected to increase.

But don't be fooled into a false sense of security if you happen to be <u>under</u> the age of 65 because the flip side of that statistic is that around 60% of those suffering from some form of heart disease are *under* age 65. It appears that heart disease does not play favorites and we are <u>all</u> at risk.

In this section you will read about some exciting new approaches to tackling heart related diseases. You will learn about a combination of all-natural extracts that one Brazilian study proved is shockingly effective at treating hypertension. You will read about the cholesterol-busting extract that was shown to dramatically reduce painful leg cramping. And you will discover the Japanese folk remedy that some researchers say may be able to dissolve deadly blood clots.

Nattokinase:
Prevent heart attack and stroke with potent enzyme that dissolves deadly blood clots in hours

The ability of blood to coagulate can be a crucial part of survival in cases of severe injury. But when blood clots occur at the wrong times, in the wrong places within the body, they can have serious—even deadly—consequences. Unfortunately, your treatment options in these circumstances are limited, and treatment must be administered quickly. Which is why prevention and knowing all of your options now—before problems occur—is crucial.

Blood clots (or thrombi) form when strands of protein called fibrin accumulate in a blood vessel. In the heart, blood clots cause blockage of blood flow to muscle tissue. If blood flow is blocked, the oxygen supply to that tissue is cut off and it eventually dies. This can result in angina and heart attacks. Clots in chambers of the heart can mobilize to the brain. In the brain, blood clots also block blood and oxygen from reaching necessary areas, which results in senility and/or stroke.

In Japan, the levels of disease and fatalities caused by blood clots are alarming. Researchers estimate that blood clots that diminish blood flow to the brain are responsible for 60 percent of all senility cases in that country.[1] Consequently, Dr. Hiroyuki Sumi—a Japanese researcher doing work at the University of Chicago's medical school—began searching for a substance that could dissolve and even prevent blood clots.

His team of researchers tested roughly 173 foods, including several types of liquor, before examining a traditional Japanese food called natto, made from boiled and fermented soybeans. The Japanese have consumed natto for centuries under the belief that it fosters cardiovascular health.

In Dr. Sumi's lab that folk remedy turned into a clinically scrutinized piece of modern medicine. He isolated an enzyme inside natto, called nattokinase, and showed that it can prevent and dissolve blood clots and may be able to safeguard people from hardened arteries, heart attack, stroke, angina, and senility.

Natto may help where modern medicine—and the human body—fall short

While the human body contains several enzymes that promote the creation of blood clots, it produces only one enzyme, plasmin, that dissolves clots, and production of that enzyme diminishes as we age.

Modern medicine includes several thrombolytic or clot-busting drugs. The leading variety is t-PA (tissue plasminogen activators), such as activase, urokinase, and streptokinase. Each year, hospitals give these drugs to more than a million stroke and heart attack patients. The treatment saves between 300,000 and 500,000 lives annually. But it's not a perfect cure. T-PAs are expensive (a dose of urokinase costs approximately US$1,500) so many patients don't receive the treatment. And the drugs' impact can be short-lived. Urokinase, for example, begins to lose effectiveness within four to 20 minutes after administration.

But when Dr. Sumi's researchers dropped natto onto an artificial thrombus (a blood clot) in a petri dish and allowed it to stand at body temperature, the blood clot gradually dissolved and disappeared completely within 18 hours. Dr. Sumi commented that nattokinase—the active enzyme in natto—showed "a potency matched by no other enzyme."[2]

The HSI network has played a key role in making this information available in North America. Through their relationship as panelists, Dr. Martin Milner of the Center for Natural Medicine in Portland, Oregon and Dr. Kouhei Makise of the Imadeqawa Makise Clinic in Kyoto, Japan were able to launch a joint research project on nattokinase and write an extensive paper on their findings. "In all my years of research as a professor of cardiovascular and pulmonary medicine, natto and nattokinase represents the most exciting new development in the prevention and treatment of cardiovascular related diseases," Dr. Milner said. "We have finally found a potent natural agent that can thin and dissolve clots effectively, with relative safety and without side effects."

**Blood clots dissolve almost 50 percent faster
with nattokinase—in as little as two hours**

Nattokinase has been the subject of 17 studies, including two small human trials.

Dr. Sumi and his colleagues induced blood clots in male dogs, then orally

---

Nattokinase Case Study Success Story
CHRONIC LEG PAIN DISAPPEARS

J. was suffering from an array of health problems including a relatively advanced case of peripheral vascular arterial disease. Her iliac artery (one of the two large arteries that supply blood to the pelvis, abdominal wall, and legs) had already been surgically bypassed several years ago when it became totally blocked and now she had another artery that was blocked. The blockage was causing her to experience the severe pain and leg weakness in her thigh and calf that is known as inter- mittent claudication. Her pain was worse at night and whenever she exerted herself. In fact, the cramps and pains she was expe- riencing every night had been disrupting her sleep for years.

A number of therapies were tried to relieve J's debilitating pain including supplements, nutritional interventions, and intra- venous EDTA treatments, but nothing seemed to work. However when J. began taking Nattokinase in July of 2002—two twice a day on an empty stomach—within just two weeks she reported that the heaviness and achiness she had been experiencing in her left leg with any sort of exertion had improved by 50 to 70 percent! The achiness in her calf muscles abated and within just two weeks J. was reporting that she was sleeping through the night with no pain. In fact, after taking Nattokinase for over 6 months J. has experienced only two episodes of the nighttime leg pain and she has reported no side effects throughout the course of therapy.

---

administered either four capsules of nattokinase (250 mg/capsule) or four placebo capsules to each dog. Angiograms (X-rays of blood vessels) revealed that the dogs who received nattokinase <u>regained normal blood circulation (free of the clot) within five hours of treatment</u>. Blood clots in the dogs who received only placebos showed no sign of dissolving in the 18 hours following treatment.

Researchers from Biotechnology Research Laboratories and JCR Pharmaceuticals Co. of Kobe, Japan, tested nattokinase's ability to dissolve a thrombus in the carotid arteries of rats. Animals treated with nattokinase regained 62 percent of blood flow, whereas those treated with plasmin regained just 15.8 percent of blood flow.[3]

Researchers from three organizations—JCR Pharmaceuticals, Oklahoma State University, and Miyazaki Medical College—tested nattokinase on 12 healthy Japanese volunteers (six men and six women, between the ages of 21 and 55). They gave the volunteers 200 grams of natto daily (before breakfast), then tracked fibrinolytic activity in the volunteers through a series of blood plasma tests. The tests indicated that the natto generated a heightened ability to dissolve blood clots: On average, the volunteers' ELT (a measure of how long it takes to dissolve a blood clot) dropped by <u>48 percent within two hours of treatment</u>, and volunteers retained an enhanced ability to dissolve blood clots for two to eight hours. As a control, researchers later fed the same amount of boiled soybeans to the same volunteers and tracked their fibrinolytic activity. The tests showed no significant change.[4]

Enhance your body's ability to fight clots without IV treatment

According to Dr. Milner, what makes nattokinase a particularly potent treatment is that it bolsters the body's natural abilities to fight blood clots in several different ways. It closely resembles plasmin and dissolves fibrin directly. In addition, it also enhances the body's production of both plasmin and other natural clot-dissolving agents, including urokinase.

In some ways, he says, nattokinase is actually superior to conventional clot-dissolving drugs. T-PAs like urokinase are only effective when taken intravenously and often fail simply because a stroke or heart attack victim's

STUDIES SUGGEST NATTO MAY PREVENT OSTEOPOROSIS

Some researchers suggest that natto might help prevent the onset of osteoporosis.

Chemical analyses of natto have revealed the fermentation process generates substantial quantities of vitamin K_2. Natto actually ranks as one of the richest sources of the vitamin. Animal studies have concluded that a diet rich in vitamin K_2 can prevent bone loss.[5] Japanese research has shown that people with osteoporosis have lower K_2 levels than people who don't have the disease.

To get the benefit of vitamin K, however, you have to eat the food version of natto. Nattokinase supplements do not contain the vitamin. If you decide to try adding natto to your diet, talk to your doctor first. Vitamin K can interfere with the normal functioning of certain medications, especially blood thinners such as Coumadin.

arteries have hardened beyond the point where they can be treated by any clot-dissolving agent. Nattokinase, however, can help prevent that hardening with an oral dose of as little as 100 mg a day.

Reduce blood pressure by 10 percent

Many Japanese have long believed that regular consumption of natto tends to lower blood pressure. Over the past several years, this belief has been substantiated by several clinical trials: In 1995, researchers reported that they had confirmed the presence of angiotensin converting enzyme (ACE) inhibitors in natto.[6] ACE causes blood vessels to narrow and blood pressure to rise. Consequently, substances that inhibit the production of ACE help lower blood pressure.

Researchers from two Japanese institutions—the Miyazaki Medical College and the Kurashiki University of Science and Arts—launched studies to test natto's impact on blood pressure in both rats and humans. They administered a single dose of natto extract (the equivalent of 25 mg of natto) into the peritoneal cavity of six male rats. On average, the rats' systolic blood pressure fell by 12.7 percent within two hours.[7]

The researchers then tested natto extract on humans. Five volunteers with high blood pressure each received the extract daily (an oral dose equivalent to 200 grams of natto) for four consecutive days. In four of the five volunteers, both systolic and diastolic blood pressure dropped. On average, systolic blood pressure fell by 10.9 percent and diastolic fell 9.7 percent.

Two companies help bring Japanese discovery to America

Since natto is traditionally a Japanese food, and one that is referred to even there as "an acquired taste," it isn't readily available in the United States. However, at least two American companies have investigated it and arranged to bring nattokinase supplements to the U.S. market. See the Source Directory starting on page 213 for ordering information. Dr. Milner has continued his research on this promising supplement. See the next page for a follow up on nattokinase.

Nattokinase Case Study Success Story
KICKING LEG PAIN, CHRONIC FATIGUE, AND HEADACHES

M. had lived for many years with a large list of medical conditions including a long standing history of chronic fatigue, varicose veins, and chronic migraine headaches. M. began to experience painful and persistant leg cramps and in January of 2003 she added a twice daily dose of two nattokinase pills to her already extensive supplement routine (which she later increased to three pills).

M. was happily surprised when not only did she see her painful leg cramps abate as her varicose veins improved, but her energy level jumped dramatically. Perhaps most startling of all her chronic migraine headaches—which had not responded to a wide variety of headache medications over the years—had completely disappeared!

NATTOKINASE FOLLOW UP

Cures for mystery diseases:
The unexpected side effects of this HSI discovery

When we first wrote about nattokinase the first shipment of this medicinal enzyme hadn't even hit the American market yet. But as new as it is here, the Japanese had long used natto—a traditional cheese-like food made by fermenting soybeans—as a remedy for vascular diseases. Then scientists discovered that natto contained an enzyme, nattokinase—and that the enzyme could break up blood clots, reduce levels of fibrin (the protein that accumulates inside blood vessels and eventually clogs them), and restore healthy circulation to diseased blood vessels. But, nattokinase was so new to the U.S. that we couldn't find physicians who could report on their experiences with it.

We thought it was time to see whether nattokinase was living up to its promise, so we called HSI Medical Adviser, Martin Milner, N.D., who has done some extensive research on nattokinase with his patients over the past few months.

Half as many "odd sensations" in just seven days

Dr. Milner told us about a patient with a history of circulatory problems who started having transient ischemic attacks (TIAs) last May. TIAs are brief episodes of reduced blood flow to isolated parts of the brain. In this patient, they resulted in frequent episodes of extremely cold hands and nose, numb lips, and odd sensations moving from the back to the front of his head. He'd been taking bromelain and Panax ginseng for several months to reduce his high fibrinogen levels and his risk of TIAs. But despite all this, he was getting steadily worse. He was about to undergo a series of IV chelation treatments when Dr. Milner convinced the man to try nattokinase instead. After just one week, his symptoms had diminished by 50 percent.

Dr. Milner saw equally dramatic improvement in a patient with severe respiratory problems. Grossly obese, hypertensive, and an early stage diabetic, the woman had episodes when she was acutely short of breath. At times, she coughed up small amounts of blood. In his clinical judgment, she was at

Nattokinase Case Study Success Story
ERASING MIGRAINE PAIN

C. who is now 64 years old had been suffering with migraine headaches since her teen years. Her headaches became even more intense frequent in the years since she entered menopause.

C. began taking nattokinase—two twice a day—in the morning and before bed. Within the first thirty days of the therapy her two to three times a week migraines had completely disappeared. Since taking nattokinase C. has experienced one episode of her pre-migraine symptoms of nausea and visual changes without ever developing actual head pain and only two actual headaches (which she suspects were brought on by drinking wine, which has been a common activator for her headaches in the past).

risk of far more serious complications—clots in the lungs, respiratory arrest, TIAs, or a stroke. A few weeks after she started nattokinase, her respiratory episodes stopped, her breathing improved, and her exercise tolerance increased.

Years of pain and fatigue begin to disappear in less than one month

To his surprise, Dr. Milner found that nattokinase could do more than address circulatory problems. It could also ease chronic diseases.

"Chronic fatigue and fibromyalgia are very difficult to treat," Dr. Milner told me, noting they are driven by multiple underlying conditions, such as high viral loads, yeast overgrowth, and hormonal imbalances. "What is usually ignored is circulatory impairment and excess clotting (hypercoagulation). It's a new thought in alternative medicine to consider that somebody is chronically fatigued because their blood clots excessively and they are not getting enough blood [and consequently, enough oxygen and nutrients] to their tissues."

In fact, Dr. Milner hadn't suspected the linkage either. But when he gave nattokinase to several patients to reduce their fibrin levels and stroke/heart attack risk, they reported back that their fibromyalgia symptoms also improved. "They experienced less muscle pain, increased energy, and more overall endurance." On average, people began feeling these benefits within seven to 30 days.

We also talked with Dr. Ralph E. Holsworth, Jr., a doctor of osteopathic medicine in Mescalaro, New Mexico. He explained a new hypothesis of disease that links circulation to a range of chronic conditions, called hyper-coagulation theory. Basically it says that any buildup of protein (or fibrin) that reduces circulation will ultimately lessen the flow of oxygen and nutrients to cells. Those deprived cells can leave the body vulnerable to a number of chronic conditions—dementia, depression, skin diseases, weakened muscles, etc. The protein buildup can also leave a person dealing with more infections (since viruses sometimes lodge in fibrin) and more pain.

"I think a lot of pain is the result of poor circulation and perfusion," Dr.

NATTOKINASE CASE STUDY SUCCESS STORY
REVERSAL OF FORTUNES; LOSS OF SENSATION RESTORED

At 63 B., who was suffering from peripheral vascular disease, was experiencing some troubling symptoms. Among his chief complaints were numbness around his lips and a feeling of coldness and loss of sensation in his hands, feet, back, head, and nose.

After starting on nattokinase twice a day—two pills in the morning and two before bed on an empty stomach—his symptoms were completely resolved within a week!

Holsworth said. "You are not getting enough oxygen to the cells so they are anaerobic and form lactic acid, which is very painful. Ask any athlete."

One long-term cancer patient he told us about had excruciating pain in her extremities due to poor circulation. Her condition left her so exhausted that she slept 14 hours a day. After three weeks on nattokinase, the pain disappeared, and she could get by on just eight hours of sleep.

Dr. Holsworth's own mother-in-law, who has lupus, was suffering from chronic pain and fibrous buildups on her skin. She even took to wearing gloves "in tropical Texas" to avoid exacerbating her symptoms. After 10 days on nattokinase, her pain and skin irritation began to ease. A few weeks later, she was able to stop taking prednisone, an anti-inflammatory derived from cortisone.

Because nattokinase effectively breaks up clots and restores circulation to diseased blood vessels, Dr. Holsworth finds it a natural alternative to prescription blood thinners, like coumadin. He's now assisting in the

---

NATTOKINASE CASE STUDY SUCCESS STORY
BREATHING EASY

K.'s medical complaints included chronic fatigue and pain, high-blood pressure, and extreme shortness of breath. In fact she was having so much trouble with her breathing that even a trip to the grocery store was exhausting and left her out of breath.

Within two and a half weeks of starting nattokinase therapy K. saw dramatic effects. Before taking the nattokinase she was unable to walk more than a half a block without extreme shortness of breath, but now she was able to easily walk an entire block without stopping and with no heavy breathing. Instead of torture, her grocery shopping trips have become pleasurable outings. Now K. reports she is walking even longer distances and has even added some light weights to her walking routine.

development of guidelines to help physicians take their patients off coumadin and put them on nattokinase. What's more, he believes that the enzyme can help diabetics and even pre-diabetics. "Because diabetes is on the rise. It's epidemic because of our S.A.D.—sad American diet. And 80 percent of people who have diabetes have heart problems." (Many diabetes medications target improved circulation to prevent heart disease as well as blood flow problems leading to amputations.)

Natto know-how: What you need for optimum success

It's important to take nattokinase carefully. It can interact with blood-thinning agents (such as coumadin, ginkgo, and antioxidants) and substances that affect platelet aggregation (including fish oil, vitamin E, and garlic). So if you're taking blood-thinning medications, you should consult your doctor before taking nattokinase and also arrange to have your fibrin levels, bleeding times, and pro-thrombin levels monitored.

You also have to take nattokinase correctly: There are some specific "rules" to follow. The capsules have a special enteric coating so they release in your small intestine, not your stomach. But they can only do that when taken on an empty stomach. (If you take them on a full stomach, they won't harm you; they just won't do you much good either.)

To date, no one has reported any negative side effects from nattokinase. One HSI member contacted us to report that a full month of nattokinase hadn't produced any noticeable effect in him. And several doctors are monitoring patients to determine exactly how much nattokinase affects fibrin levels over time.

All these dramatic healing benefits for just "pennies a day"

One nattokinase supplement is available directly through Dr, Milner. And Dr. Milner provides telephone consultations to individuals who need information on how to use nattokinase effectively and safely. (See the Source Directory starting on page 213 for further information.)

But you don't have to buy supplements in order to benefit from nattokinase.

"I tell my patients that they can make natto for pennies a day," Dr. Holsworth said. (You can find directions for making your own natto online at www.gaia21.net/natto.)

In addition to saving money, you can actually get added health benefits by eating the whole food. Natto contains nutrients that also help fight cancer and osteoporosis.

For a preventive dose, simply eat 3 1/4 tablespoons of natto each day. For a therapeutic dose, eat 6 1/2 tablespoons.

"The ironic thing," Dr. Holsworth noted, "is that when we occupied Japan after the war, we said that natto was unsanitary because of its smell and preparation. Because of that false presumption, we forbade the Japanese from using it. Now the food that we banned is coming into the United States and we are touting it as a medicinal food."

References

[1]   "Interview with Doctor of Medicine Hiroyuki Sumi," Japan Bio Science Laboratory Co. Ltd.

[2]   Acta Haematol, 84: 139-43, 1990

[3]   Biol Pharm Bull, 18(10): 1.387-91, 1995 Oct

[4]   Acta Haematol, 84: 139-43, 1990

[5]   Plant Foods Hum Nutr, 47(1): 39-47, 1995 Jan

[6]   JTTAS, 1995

[7]   ibid

CHAPTER 29

Policicsanol:

Sugar cane extract rivals popular cholesterol-lowering drugs, without dangerous side effects

Amid reports of health problems and deaths caused by statin drugs, we've learned that an extract of a commercial crop—sugar cane—can lower cholesterol just as effectively.

As we've told you over the past five years, cholesterol isn't the primary cause of heart disease...homocysteine levels are. Nevertheless, cholesterol *does* play an important role in coronary health, and any good program for reversing heart disease must address that as well. So you can imagine how excited we were when our researchers discovered that a sugar cane extract could *dramatically* reduce cholesterol levels.

While it's drawn from the same plant that produces table sugar, policosanol doesn't affect blood sugar levels when ingested. Cuban scientists, however, have discovered that it can have a cholesterol-reducing effect[1] without creating the uncomfortable and even dangerous side effects associated with statin drugs.[2,3] Statin drugs lower elevated cholesterol by limiting cholesterol production in the liver, but they also have side effects ranging from heartburn to potentially fatal cases of muscle breakdown (see the box on page 198). This widely prescribed class of drugs—statin sales topped $14 billion last year—includes the brand names Lipitor, Lescol, Zocor, Mevacor, Pravachol, Prevastatin, and Baycol (which was recalled after being linked to over 40 deaths).

In several studies that compared both cholesterol-lowering methods, policosanol surpassed the performance of statin-drug therapy. One Cuban study compared the effects of policosanol to Pravastatin on patients who had elevated cholesterol levels and were considered to be at high risk for coronary disease. Patients took 10 mg of either policosanol or Pravastatin with their dinners for 8 weeks. The group taking statins saw their LDL levels fall by 15.6 percent and their total cholesterol by 11.8 percent. But those in the policosanol group exceeded those numbers, and dropped their LDL levels by 19.3 percent and their total cholesterol by 13.9 percent. **The HDL levels of the statin test subjects remained the same, while the <u>policosanol group increased their HDL levels by 15.7 percent</u>.** Because HDL cholesterol aids in the removal of fat from arterial walls, an increase in these levels is beneficial.

Thousands of people struggle with cholesterol problems, and the chance

---

YOU CAN'T LIVE WITHOUT CHOLESTEROL

Cholesterol is a fat and is essential to life. In fact, it's so important that your body manufactures it instead of being wholly dependent on dietary sources. Your liver makes about 80 percent of your cholesterol, which is used in a number of bodily functions, including:

- the movement and absorption of fatty acids
- the manufacture of vitamin D on the skin's surface
- the production of sex and adrenal hormones, including estrogen, testosterone, cortisone and DHEA (dehydroepiandosterone)
- the creation of fatty covers around nerve fibers

Cholesterol is found mostly in egg yolks and animal fat. If you eat too much cholesterol, your liver makes less of it. Eat too little, and your liver makes up the deficit.

Cholesterol is measured as a whole as well as by its components, which are LDL (low-density lipoprotein), or "bad" cholesterol, and HDL (high-density lipoprotein), or "good" cholesterol. Even if your total cholesterol count is below 200 mg/dL, which is generally thought to be good, having a low HDL level (less than 40 mg/dL) or a high LDL level (above 130 mg/dL) is believed to increase the risk of vascular disease. Ideally LDL should be less than 100 mg/dl.

---

of developing high cholesterol increases as we age. As we grow older, our hormone levels drop, making it easier for cholesterol levels to rise in our bodies. Researchers believe policosanol may be a safe method of reducing and regulating LDL. In a clinical trial involving 244 post-menopausal women with high cholesterol, researchers first attempted to bring down elevated lipid levels through six weeks of a standard lipid-lowering diet. When this proved unsuccessful, they gave the women 5 mg of policosanol daily for 12 weeks, then 10 mg daily for another 12 weeks. Researchers found that the supplement was effective in significantly lowering LDL levels (25.2 percent) and total cholesterol (16.7 percent). In addition, the women experienced a **29.3 percent increase in HDL levels.**[4]

Extract relieves painful leg cramps

One of the common—and debilitating—side effects of high cholesterol is a syndrome known as intermittent claudication—a cramping pain in the calves. This is often linked to poor circulation and the presence of arterial fat deposits (atherosclerosis). Intermittent claudication occurs only during certain times, such as after walking. Removal of arterial fat deposits has been found to decrease claudication.

Researchers at the Medical Surgical Research Center in Havana, Cuba tested policosanol patients who suffered from moderately severe intermittent claudication. In this two-year long study, 56 patients were randomly assigned to receive either policosanol or a placebo. Researchers determined if the policosanol was relieving the claudication by conducting treadmill walking tests on each subject before the study and again 6, 12, 18, and 24 months after beginning treatment. Although both test groups showed some progress during the interim tests, the final results indicated that policosanol had a significant benefit for sufferers of intermittent claudication. After two years of treatment, patients in the placebo group were able to walk a maximum of .15 miles while the group taking policosanol could walk .40 miles before having to stop. The **21 people taking policosanol increased their walking distance by at least 50 percent**. Only five members of the placebo group showed a similar improvement.[5]

And it's possible that policosanol could do more than alleviate the risk of heart disease, circulatory problems and other ailments commonly associated with high cholesterol...

STATIN DRUGS: ARE THE DANGEROUS HEALTH RISKS WORTH IT?

Statin drugs, such as lovastatin, were originally derived from red yeast rice, though the current base of most is synthetic. Their cholesterol-lowering abilities aren't questioned, but the baggage that comes with reduced cholesterol is significant. The side effects of statins include the following:[7]

- Gas
- Stomach pain or cramps and/or upset stomach
- Diarrhea and/or constipation
- Heartburn
- Headache and/or dizziness
- Blurred vision
- Rash or itching

In addition to the conditions above, which are the most common side effects, statins can produce seriously adverse effects, such as rhabdomyolysis. This disorder is characterized by wasting muscles and causes muscle cell contents to be released into the bloodstream. As the tissue deteriorates, organs may fail and cause death. In fact, the statin drug Baycol was recalled this August, because it caused a higher rate of rhabdomyolysis than most other statin drugs and was linked to at least 40 deaths. Nevertheless, the muscle-wasting disorder can still attack those who take other statin products. Another serious side effect of statin-drug use is liver damage. In studies involving statin drugs, liver enzymes, such as alanine aminotransferase, are routinely measured to determine if the drugs have caused any liver damage.

A possible defense against Alzheimer's

Dora M. Kovacs, Ph.D., a researcher at Massachusetts General Hospital, recently received a $200,000 research grant to study the side effects of cholesterol on the development of Alzheimer's Disease (AD). She found that even normal levels of cholesterol may increase the risk of senility-causing plaques and neurofibrillary tangles in the brain, which are associated with the development and progress of AD.[6]

Dr. Kovacs' research is focusing on the development of drugs that inhibit the production of ACAT, an enzyme that enables cholesterol and other lipids (fats) to enter cells and form solid lipid droplets there. Those droplets can hinder the normal functioning of the cell. They can also increase amyloid beta production, which is associated with the progress of mind-robbing plaques and tangles. When lipid droplet levels increase, amyloid beta production increases...and so does the risk of Alzheimer's.

Dr. Kovacs and her research team beleive that ACAT-inhibiting drugs are the keys to halting the process of cholesterol and lipid buildup that results in AD. But the related research is in its early stages. Dr. Kovacs plans, but has not yet started, to test ACAT inhibitors on mice specially bred to have AD. Other researchers have developed a potentially safe class of ACAT inhibitors to treat atherosclerosis. But it may be another five to 10 years before this family of drugs is thoroughly developed, tested, and made available to the public.

There may be an alternative therapy available right now, however. In an interview with Emma Hitt, Ph.D. for the Reuters news service, Dr. Kovacs indicated that several studies have shown that patients who take statin drugs have lower rates of AD and other types of dementia. Cholesterol-lowering statins do not appear to hinder the ACAT enzyme, but the act of maintaining low cholesterol levels lowers the risk of dementia.

Since statin drugs can induce serious side effects, policosanol may prove to be a better alternative. In double-blind trials, policosanol produced mild, short-term side effects—such as insomnia, headache, diarrhea, nervousness, and weight loss—in less than one percent of test subjects. So policosanol may prove to be an efficacious mind-saver as well as a life-saver.

Caution: Researchers warn that policosanol can interact with blood-thinning drugs. So if you try policosanol (after consulting your doctor), your dose of blood-thinning medication may have to be adjusted with careful medical monitoring.

If you would like more information on purchasing policosanol, see the Source Directory starting on page 213.

If you're already taking cholesterol-lowering drugs or being treated for any other health condition, you should consult with your doctor before trying policosanol or discontinuing any prescription drug.

LIPID OXIDATION CAN INCREASE CARDIOVASCULAR DISEASE

If you're not already taking antioxidant supplements, policosanol can offer you a double benefit. While it controls your cholesterol levels, it can also prevent lipid oxidation—a mutation of fat cells that heightens an individual's risk of cardiovascular disease.

At the Center of Natural Products in Havana, Cuba, researchers conducted a double-blind, randomized, placebo-controlled trial on 69 healthy subjects to determine if policosanol supplementation could reduce the markers indicative of LDL oxidation. After eight weeks of supplementation, researchers found that policosanol could decrease oxidative markers and postpone the onset of oxidation by 57 percent when compared to subjects taking a placebo.[8]

References

[1] Arch Med Res, 29(1):21-4, 1998

[2] Rev Med Chil, 127(3):286-94, 1999

[3] Int J Clin Pharmacol Res, 19(4):117-27, 1999

[4] Gynecol Endocrinol, 14(3):187-95, 2000

[5] Angiology, 52(2):115-25, 2001

[6] www.ahaf.org/alzdis/ research/awards_body.htm

[7] www.drugdigest.org

[8] Br J Pharmacol, 50(3):255-62, 2000

C H A P T E R **30**

Pressure FX:

Yale-trained scientist develops powerful combination of natural extracts. Hypertension treatment proves 88 percent effective in Brazilian study

Sometimes a promising treatment arises from the strangest circumstances. Recently, the discovery of a new hormone and the contents of a stray pamphlet from Vancouver's Chinatown were the unlikely components that led a Yale-trained pharmacologist to a discovery that could eliminate your need for prescription hypertension drugs.

Hypertension, or high blood pressure, is one of the most common forms of cardiovascular disease in North America. Roughly 25 percent of the population has it, and the condition can lead to serious medical problems, including stroke, renal failure, arteriosclerosis (hardening of the arteries), heart attack, and congestive heart failure. Odds are, if you or someone you know has been diagnosed with high blood pressure, the doctor has recommended certain mainstays of conventional cardiovascular treatment—such as dietary modifications and prescription drugs. But this new discovery may be able to dramatically enhance the positive effects of dietary changes in order to regulate blood pressure, and potentially reduce or even eliminate the need for prescription drugs in people with salt-sensitive hypertension.

Canadian lab uncovers calcium's role in high blood pressure

For years, physicians believed that hypertension was a single disease with an unknown cause. Up until the 1980s, roughly 90 percent of all cases were listed as "essential hypertension," meaning the cause of the heightened blood pressure was unknown.

Eventually, however, researchers realized that significant numbers of hypertension patients shared certain characteristics. A particularly large number (about 40 percent of all cases) suffered from salt-sensitive blood pressure along with low levels of a substance called renin, a kidney enzyme that plays a major role in easing high blood pressure. They also shared a peculiar condition—they all had low blood calcium levels but elevated levels of parathyroid hormone (the hormone responsible for maintaining healthy blood calcium levels). Researchers speculated that some compound in the body was inhibiting the normal function of the hormone and began searching for it.

At the University of Alberta in western Canada, Dr. Peter Pang—a Yale-trained pharmacologist and head of U of A's department of physiology—led a group of researchers in an effort to find the cause of this type of hypertension. Through a series of tests on laboratory animals, they determined that a second hormone produced by the parathyroid gland was depressing calcium levels in the blood and causing high blood pressure.[1] They named the hormone parathyroid hypertensive factor or PHF. Essentially, PHF causes calcium, which should circulate in the bloodstream, to build up inside cells. These calcium-heavy cells place increased pressure on arteries which increases blood pressure inside the arteries. In fact, one of the major categories of prescription drugs used to treat hypertension are calcium channel blockers that reduce the amount of calcium ions passing into the cells.

Once they realized what was causing the "unexplained" 40 percent of all hypertension cases—and high intracellular calcium, scientists had a foundation to search for new remedies.

Through his company, CV Technologies—a research and development company focused on using traditional Chinese and herbal medicines to produce modern nutraceuticals—Dr. Pang developed Pressure FX specifically to address hypertension caused by PHF. Its components are unusual, and the clinical research behind them is still sparse. But Dr. Pang asserts that it is an effective treatment for salt-sensitive hypertension, and his claim has been backed up by several studies.

Tibetan caterpillar mushroom helps stimulate drop in blood pressure

Practitioners of traditional Chinese medicine have used Cordyceps Sinensis for centuries to improve lung and kidney function, to suppress coughs, and to regulate blood coagulation. According to reports of traditional usage, it has helped ease respiratory diseases, treat arrhythmias, and reduce high blood pressure.[2] Cordyceps, one of the two components of Pressure FX, is a fungus found in the highlands of China, Tibet, and Nepal (at elevations ranging from 3,500 to 10,000 feet above sea level). It is commonly known as caterpillar mushroom.

Researchers at the University of Alberta tested Cordyceps' potential for lowering blood pressure by injecting various solutions (dosage ranged from 0.03mg/kg to 10 mg/kg) into anesthetized rats, then measuring the blood pressure in a tail artery. The experiments produced dose-dependent reductions in blood pressure. However, the effect was often fleeting—beginning within 15 seconds of treatment and ending barely a minute later.[3]

Scientists at the National Research Institute of Chinese Medicine in Taiwan achieved better results using higher doses of Cordyceps. They injected anesthetized rats with doses of 8, 16, 24, or 32 mg/kg. Not only did the treatment reduce blood pressure in a dose dependent manner, but the effect continued for 45 minutes.[4]

A cancer treatment's hidden heart potential uncovered in Chinatown

Shark cartilage, the other component of Pressure FX, is more widely known for its ability to inhibit the growth of tumors. And even Dr. Pang admits that it's not the first thing he would expect to include in a hypertension formula. "I would have never suspected something like shark cartilage, or added it to my mainstream research," he commented, "but serendipity plays a role in science."

Dr. Pang was in the midst of searching for a treatment for PHF-induced hypertension when a friend showed him a pamphlet he'd found in Vancouver's Chinatown describing shark cartilage's potential for treating diabetes, colon cancer, and breast cancer—conditions that Dr. Pang had already linked to excess intracellular calcium and possibly to PHF. With this knowledge as a base, he decided to test shark cartilage for hypertension.

Pang's researchers injected shark cartilage into spontaneously hypertensive rats. When they did, the animals' blood pressure dropped. The treatment also helped normalize the rate of calcium buildup in the animals' cells.[5] The researchers also tested shark cartilage on rats with normal blood pressure. When they injected the healthy rats with PHF, the rats' blood pressure rose. However, when they gave the rats an injection of shark cartilage first, then gave them PHF, the rats' blood pressure didn't rise.

Although the exact mechanism that enables shark cartilage to control blood pressure isn't known, Dr. Pang theorizes that "it is possible—I must stress possible—that shark cartilage contains something that antagonizes PHF."

High blood pressure corrected in 88 percent of patients

Since results from intravenous applications of nutrients and therapies are often different from those obtained by oral administration, more research on shark cartilage's effects on hypertension when taken orally was necessary. A group of Brazilian physicians tested the actual supplement form of Pressure FX in a clinical trial involving 102 hypertensive patients (74 with mild hypertension, 28 with moderate hypertension).[6] The researchers tracked each patient's condition for three to 12 months. Each subject took one to three Pressure FX capsules daily. Before they started taking the supplement, however, subjects received other forms of treatment. They followed researchers' instructions to modify their lifestyle, including instructions to increase their consumption of fruit, vegetables, and legumes; to decrease their consumption of foods linked to lipid oxidation; and to take calcium, magnesium, and potassium supplements (which are commonly recommended to ease high blood pressure). In addition, 87 subjects received chelation therapy (10 to 20 treatments each).

The results were dramatic. Before the study began, the group's mean blood pressure was 171.42 over 107.95. After treatment it was 126.13 over 83.36. The Brazilian researchers reported that between 50 and 60 percent of subjects responded to the lifestyle modifications and mineral supplementation alone. When Pressure FX was added to the treatment regimen, the number of subjects showing significantly reduced blood pressure jumped to 88 percent.

Of the 84 subjects who were taking hypertension drugs prior to the study, 63 were able to stop medication and maintain normal blood pressure with Pressure FX.

Pressure FX eases hypertension when other treatments fail

In a recent article in the *Townsend Newsletter for Doctors and Patients*, Nelson Kraucak, M.D., ABFP, reported on his experience using Pressure FX at the Life Family Practice Center for Complementary Medicine in Lady Lake, Florida. Dr. Kraucak advised patients who weren't responding to other treatments (such as magnesium, L-carnitine, and coenzyme Q10) to take

---

COULD DIABETES AND CANCER BE THE RESULT OF "EXCESSIVE PHF SYNDROME?"

Although researchers originally linked PHF to hypertension only, subsequent research has suggested that excessive amounts of parathyroid hypertensive factor may contribute to other diseases.

"By the time we got the mechanism of PHF studied, we realized that it was not just a hypertension hormone. It was an intracellular calcium regulating hormone," says Dr. Pang. "That is very, very significant, because a lot of diseases and health problems are related to abnormal cellular calcium regulation."

People with type II diabetes often have heightened cellular calcium levels—a situation that disables their insulin receptors and exacerbates the disease. Intracellular calcium also affects mitosis (cell division), and very preliminary research suggests that PHF may play a role in some cancers. A small-scale study conducted by Dr. Pang and his associates showed that 60 percent of breast cancer patients and 70 percent of colon cancer patients have elevated PHF levels.[7]

Dr. Pang is currently investigating PHF's links to other diseases, and the possibility that PHF treatments could prove effective against ailments other than hypertension.

---

one capsule of Pressure FX three times a day. He reported the treatment was effective in 65 percent of his patients.

The twists of fate that led Dr. Pang to develop this unique formula could mean a world of difference for the millions of people suffering from hypertension. Pressure FX appears to be a safe, effective treatment for regulating blood pressure levels. CV Technologies assures us it conducts assays on each batch of supplements to ensure they remain consistent.

Ordering information for Pressure FX is listed in the Source Directory starting on page 213.

References
[1]   Blood Press, 3(3): 147, 1994

[2]   www.china-window.com

[3]   J Chin Med, 7(2): 153-167, 1996

[4]   Life Sci, 66(14): 1,369-76, 2000

[5]   Townsend Letter, 223/224: 82-84, 2002

[6]   ibid.

[7]   www.herbtech.com

CHAPTER 31

TheaChol:

You don't need expensive–and dangerous– statin drugs! Protect your heart with this safe, natural, and affordable alternative

You know that tea can be good for your heart. But did you know that the phytochemicals in tea can lower your cholesterol levels by as much as 27 points?

It's true. And according to research, a drop like that could reduce your risk of heart disease more than 30 percent.[1]

There's just one problem. To realize those benefits, you'd have to drink as many as *57 cups of tea every day*. And you'd have to drink both green tea and black tea throughout the day to get the full impact.

Still interested? We know we wouldn't be. But luckily, that's not the end of the story.

Scientists have found a way to deliver tea's powerful active ingredients without getting bogged down in cup counts. Even better, they've found a way to combine the best of green tea and the best of black tea, to offer the greatest benefits of both. These discoveries have produced impressive results—in some cases, results comparable to those seen with statin drugs—but at a much lower cost and without scary side effects.

Green or black? It's all in the flavonoids...

For centuries, people have been drinking tea. And for several decades now, science has recognized the heart-healthy benefits of the habit. Research shows that the more tea people drink, the lower their cholesterol—and more importantly, the lower the incidence of cardiovascular disease.[2,3]

For these benefits, we can thank *flavonoids*, plant-pigment molecules found in the leaves of the tea plant, *camellia sinensis*. Depending on how they are prepared, these leaves can end up as either green or black tea, each providing its own type of flavonoids.

Green tea is made from the dried leaves of *camellia sinensis*, and is rich in flavonoids called *catechins*. To make black tea, the leaves are fermented; during the fermentation process the molecules in catechins rearrange to form polymer flavonoids called *theaflavins*.

Both types of flavonoids offer powerful health benefits, and not just for the heart (see the box below for other positive benefits of tea). Although there's been some debate about which type of tea is best, it's really not an issue of one vs. the other. The catechins in green tea and the theaflavins in black tea both offer unique benefits.

Animal studies have shown that catechins can reduce intestinal absorption of cholesterol and increase the excretion of fat and cholesterol through the feces.[4,5] Green tea catechins can also reduce the concentration of cholesterol in the livers of mice, and can even increase the LDL binding activity of human liver cells, lowering circulating plasma levels of low-density lipoprotein (a.k.a. "bad cholesterol"). Other animal studies have shown that black tea theaflavins can also increase fecal excretion of fat and cholesterol.[8-10]

These studies—combined with centuries of anecdotal evidence and data from observational studies—provide impressive support of tea flavonoids' cholesterollowering power. But one question remained unanswered—until now.

Just imagine: if tea catechins and theaflavins can exert this much influence individually, what would happen if we could put them together? That's just what a team of scientists in China asked themselves. They hypothesized that combining theaflavins and catechins would increase each flavonoid's individual power exponentially. And guess what—they were right.

In just 12 weeks, total cholesterol levels decreased more than 11 percent!

The scientists recruited 240 men and women with mild to moderate hypercholesterolemia (high cholesterol), which they defined as LDL levels between 130 and 190 mg/dL. (Most health authorities recommend keeping LDL levels below 130 mg/dL.) After baseline assessments were collected, the participants were blindly divided into two groups: one group took a placebo each morning, while the other took a capsule containing 75 mg of theaflavins and 300 mg of green tea flavonoids, including catechins. The participants followed this routine for 12 weeks, and had their blood levels rechecked at weeks 4 and 12.

Here's what the researchers found: after just four weeks, the intervention group's total cholesterol was down by nearly seven percent, and their LDL

FLAVONOIDS AREN'T JUST FOR THE HEART
RESEARCH SHOWS THESE PHYTOCHEMICALS IMPART
A WHOLE HOST OF HEALTHY BENEFITS

Scientists aren't only interested in tea flavonoids for their cholesterollowering power. Other research has shown that tea may also have the following properties:

- Antibacterial
- Antioxidant
- Antiviral
- Anticarcinogenic
- Antimutagenic

In a study just published in the journal *Carcinogenesis*, researchers at the Linus Pauling Institute showed that moderate consumption of tea (about three cups a day) can protect against colon cancer about as well as the prescription non-steroidal anti-inflammatory drug sulindac.[6] Other studies have shown tea's anticarcinogenic and antimutagenic effects against prostate cancer and gastric cancer. And in research at the U.S. Department of Agriculture, scientists found that the polyphenols in tea, particularly theaflavins, catechins, and another flavonoid called epicatechin gallate, may also help increase insulin activity.[7] In laboratory tests, tea increased insulin activity 15-fold—a discovery that might help address the rising tide of insulin resistance.

---

decreased almost 10 percent! After 12 weeks, the numbers were even more impressive: total cholesterol levels in the flavonoid group were down more than 11 percent, with LDL levels down more than 16 percent. At the same time, the placebo group saw total and LDL cholesterol levels stay the same or creep up. Even better, none of the participants in the intervention group experienced any negative side effects from the flavonoid supplement.[11]

Cholesterol isn't everything...but it's still important

At HSI, we've talked a lot about how cholesterol is not the be-all, end-all of heart health. We still maintain that position; after all, even the mainstream is now admitting to the importance of other heart health markers like homocysteine and c-reactive protein. But the fact remains that cholesterol levels, particularly LDL cholesterol levels, are still an important part of the whole picture. Observational studies have shown that for every 10-point-reduction in cholesterol level, your risk of heart attack or other major cardiovascular event falls as much as 15 percent.[12]

If you know your levels are too high, chances are your doctor has talked to you about taking statin drugs. But we all know the problems inherent with that approach—astronomical prices and a laundry list of frightening side effects, including liver damage, sexual dysfunction, peripheral neuropathy, and vitamin deficiency.

But now this research provides us all with another option: a safe, natural, affordable supplement that delivers the cholesterol-lowering power of flavonoids in one capsule—without having to drink gallons of tea.

Confidential access for HSI makes you the first to benefit

The supplement is called TheaChol. It is the exact same formulation of tea flavonoids used in the Chinese study that saw such impressive results. And as you read this, you're among the first people in the world to have access to this product—and this information.

That's right: as we write this, the Chinese study quoted above is being prepared for presentation at a large medical association convention, and for publication in a major medical journal in 2003. HSI received confidential access to the research before it even hit the presses. That means you're learning about the power of this theaflavin enriched green tea extract before most mainstream doctors will even get around to reading about it (if they ever do). You have one of the first opportunities to put the cholesterol-lowering power of TheaChol to work for you today.

By taking just one TheaChol capsule per day, you'll get 375 mg of thea-flavins and other tea flavonoids—the equivalent of 25 to 57 cups of tea. And you can get a full month's supply of TheaChol for less than half the cost of a month's worth of statin drugs. (See the Source Directory starting on page 213 for complete ordering information.)

TheaChol really provides the best of all possible worlds: all the flavonoid power of both green and black tea without having to drink gallons of it AND it offers significant cholesterol-lowering effects without having to incur the costs or risks of statins.

It is important to note that a study published in 2002 suggests that stopping statin therapy "cold turkey" can result in a three percent increase in the risk of death and non-fatal heart attacks.[13] So if you have been diagnosed with acute coronary disease and are currently taking statin drugs, speak with your doctor before discontinuing your medication to try TheaChol.

References

[1] Prev Med, 21(4):546-553, 1992 Jul

[2] Prev Med, 21(4):546-553, 1992 Jul

[3] Arch Intern Med 1999, 159(18):2170-2174, Oct 11

[4] Biochim Biophys Acta, 1127(2):141-146, 1992 Jul 29

[5] J Nutr Sci Vitaminol, 44(2):337-342, 1998 Apr

[6] Carcinogenesis, 24(2):263-267, 2003 Feb

[7] J Agric Food Chem, 50(24):7182-7186, 2002 Nov

[8] In Vivo, 14(4):481-484, 2000 July-Aug

[9] J Agric Food Chem, 49(11):5639-5645, 2001 Nov

[10] J Nutr Sci Vitaminol, 44(2):337-342, 1998 Apr

[11] Abstract #1057-146 presented American College of Cardiology, Chicago, 2003 March

[12] Circulation, 97:946-952, 1998 March

[13] Circulation, 105(12):1446-52, 2002 March

Source Directory

Many of the remedies discussed in *Underground Cures* are so cutting edge that they may not be readily available in health food stores or retail outlets in your area. As a service to our readers we have identified (whenever possible) a high-quality and reliable source for the products discussed in this book.

Please note: Agora Health Books verified all product information when this book was written; however, pricing and availability can change by the time your book is delivered.

Section I
Breakthroughs in Conquering Cancer

Chapter 1

Agaricus Blazei Murrill (ABM) Mushroom

VirtuVites
5092 Buttercup Dr.
Castle Rock, CO 80104
Tel: (800) 332-5069 or (303) 814-6980
Fax: (303) 814-0187
www.virtuvites.com

Chapter 2

**Glycoalkaloid cream
(ask for SkinAnswer)**

Compassionet
P.O. Box 710
Saddle River, NJ, 07458
Tel: (800) 510-2010, Ext. 474 or
Tel: (201) 236-3900, Ext. 474
Fax: (201) 236-0090
www.compassionet.com

Chapter 3

Fucoidan

American BioSciences
560 Bradley Parkway
Blauvelt, NY 10913
Tel: (888) 884-7770 or (845) 727-0800
Fax: (845) 727-0864

Chapter 4

Guacatonga

Raintree Nutrition, Inc.
10609 Metric Blvd.
Austin, TX 78758
Tel: (800) 780-5902 or (512) 833-5006
Fax: (512) 833-5454
www.rain-tree.com

Chapter 5

Larreastat™

Robert A. Sinnott, Ph.D.
Larreacorp, Ltd.
P.O. Box 6598
Chandler, AZ 85246-6598
Tel: (800) 682-9448 or (480) 963-7310
Fax: (480) 659-0125
www.larreacorp.com
To learn more about Larreastat, you may e-mail Dr. Sinnott directly at rasinnott@yahoo.com.

Section II
Anti-aging Answers

Chapter 6
AstaFactor
Aquasearch, Inc.
73-4460 Queen Kaahumanu
Highway, Suite 110
Kailuakona, HI 96740
Tel: (800) 480-6515 or (808) 327-4020

Chapter 7
Natural Dismutase Compound
Health Research Associates
P.O. Box 820083
Portland, OR 97215
Tel: (877) 635-7070 or (503) 239-0009
*(voicemail will be answered by Dr.
Robert Doughton)*
Fax: (503) 239-0008

Chapter 8
Energy Kampo (Juzen-taiho-to)
Willner Chemists
100 Park Avenue
New York, NY 10017
Tel: (800) 633-1106 or (212) 682-2817
Fax: (212) 682-6192
www.willner.com/honso.htm

Chapter 9
Clavo Huasca
Raintree Nutrition, Inc.
10609 Metric Blvd.
Austin, TX 78758
Tel: (800) 780-5902 or (512) 833-5006
Fax: (512) 833-5414
www.rain-tree.com

Chapter 10
Liver Kampo
BenSalem Naturals
371 Dartmouth Center
Bensalem, PA 19020-8204
Tel: (215) 638-0627
www.bnatural.com

Liver Kampo
Willner Chemists
100 Park Avenue
New York, NY 10017
Tel: (800) 633-1106 or (212) 682-2817
Fax: (212) 682-6192
www.willner.com/honso.htm

Chapter 11
MindCare
Himalaya USA
10440 Westoffice Dr.
Houston, TX 77042
Tel: (800) 869-4640 or (713) 863-1622
Fax: (800) 577-6930
www.himalyausa.com

Section III
Breathing Free

Chapter 12
Buteyko Home Education Kit
Buteyko Asthma
2507 Brewster Road
Indianapolis, IN 46268
Tel: (877) 278-4623 or (317) 824-0328

Chapter 13
Serrapeptase
Optimal Health Resources/PCE &
Associates
550 Kane Ct., Suite 100
Oviedo, FL 32765
Tel: (888) 727-6388 or (407) 366-8208
Fax: (407) 366-3343

Section IV
Super Immunity Boosters

Chapter 14
CellAid
Herbaceuticals, Inc.
630 Airpark Road
Napa, CA 94558
Tel: (800) 784-8212 or (707) 259-6266

Chapter 15
Kan Jang
IHerb
600 E. Fig Avenue
Monrovia, CA 91016
Tel: (888) 792-0028 or (626) 358-5678
Fax: (626) 303-7275
www.iHerb.com

Chapter 16
TryptoZen
Optimal Health Resources
550 Kane Court, Suite 100
Oviedo, FL 32765
Tel: (888) 727-6388 or (407) 977-5689
Fax: (407) 366-3343

Suanzaorentang Formula (wild jujube)
J-Lin Alternative Healing
45 Popham Road, Suite E
Scarsdale, NY 10583
Tel & Fax: (914) 725-7557
www.powertoheal.com
*(For more information on J-Lin
Alternative Healing. Products are not
currently sold on website.)*

Relora
BioBalance International
1608 Michael Lane
Pacific Palisades, CA 90272
Tel: (888) 246-4416 or (310) 459-9866
Fax: (310) 459-9466
www.natural-chemistry.com

Chapter 17
ViraMedx and Shingle-EEZE
Merix Health Care Products
18 E. Dundee Rd., 3-204
Barrington, IL 60010
Tel: (800) 224-4024 or (847) 277-1111
www.viramedx.com

Chapter 18
Zen
Optimal Health Resources
550 Kane Court, Suite 100
Oviedo, FL, 32765
Tel: (888) 727-6388 or (407) 977-5689
Fax: (407) 366-3343

Adrenal stress profile testing (cortisol x4)
North Bay Diagnostics
13606 S. West Bay Shore Drive
P.O. Box 4150
Traverse City, MI 49685-4150
Tel: (888) 689-8378 or (231) 922-2295
Fax: (231) 922-2274

Section V
Powerful Pain Relief

Chapter 19

**Foundation Formula &
Renew Formula**

Forever Well
P.O. Box 14653
Reading, PA 19612
Tel: (800) 619-5969 or (610) 374-5258
Fax: (419) 781-3161
www.foreverwell.com

Chapter 20

JointCare

Himalaya USA
10440 Westoffice Dr.
Houston, Texas 77042
Tel: (800) 869-4640 or (713) 863-1622
Fax: (800) 577-6930
www.himalayausa.com

Chapter 21

Lumbricus Tonic (Earth Dragon)

Nutricology
30806 Santana Street
Hayward, CA 94544
Tel: (800) 782-4274 or (510) 487-8526

Chapter 22

Nexrutine™

Solanova
7110 Redwood Blvd., Suite A
Novato, CA 94945
Tel: (800) 200-0456 or (415) 898-1704
Fax: (415) 898-1666
www.solanova.com

Chapter 23

Potter's Acidosis

Potter's Herbal Medicines
Leyland Mill Lane
Wigan, Lanc WN1 2SB,
United Kingdom
Tel: 011-44-1942-405100
Fax: 011-44-1942-820255
www.goodnessdirect.co.uk,
www.herbal-direct.com,
www.academyhealth.com

Chapter 24

UriCare

Himalaya USA
10440 Westoffice Dr.
Houston, TX 77042
Tel: (800) 869-4640 or (713) 863-1622
Fax: (800) 577-6930
www.himalayausa.com

Section VI
Fight Diabetes & Win

Chapter 25

Glucotor

Healing America
426 Salem Drive
Owensboro, KY 42303
Fax: (270) 688-8344
www.northernnutrition.healingamer-ica.com

Chapter 26

Pancreas Support and Chanca Piedra

Raintree Nutrition, Inc.
10609 Metric Boulevard
Austin, TX 78758
Tel: (800) 780-5902 or (512) 833-5006
Fax: (512) 833-5414
www.rain-tree.com

Chapter 27

Sugar Blocker

Harmony Company
P.O. Box 93
Northvale, NJ 07647
Tel: (800) 422-5518 or (860) 426-1518

Section VII
Heart Healthy Solutions

Chapter 28

Nattokinase

Center for Natural
Medicine Dispensary
1330 S.E. 39th Ave.
Portland, OR 97214
Tel: (888) 305-4288 or (503) 232-0475
Fax: (503) 232-7751
www.cnm-inc.com
If you are thinking about trying natto-kinase but would like to speak with a physician first, HSI medical advisor Marty Milner, N.D., is available for phone consultations.
Please call (503) 232-1100 to schedule an appointment.

Nattokinase

Tahoma Clinic Dispensary
801 SW 16th
Renton, WA 98055
Tel: (888) 893-6878 or (425) 264-0051
Fax: (425) 264-0058
www.tahoma-clinic.com

Chapter 29

Policosanol

Optimal Health Resources
550 Kane Court, Suite A
Oviedo, Florida 32765
Tel: (888) 727-6388 or (407) 366-8208
Fax: (407) 366-3343

Chapter 30

Pressure FX

Optimal Health Resources
550 Kane Court, Suite 100
Oviedo, FL 32765
Tel: (888) 727-6388 or (407) 366-8208
(this number is answered by PCE & Associates)
Fax: (407) 366-3343

Chapter 31

TheaChol

NorthStar Nutritionals
P.O. Box 925
Frederick, MD 21705
Tel: (800) 311-1950 or (203) 699-4438
and ask for Order Code NSNTEA

APPENDIX **B**

Index

– A –

Acidophilus, 145–48

Actinic keratoses (AK), 10, 12

Agaricus blazei murrill (ABM) mushroom, 3–7

Age spots, 10–11

Age-related ailments, 32, 37

Age-related macular degeneration (ARMD), 31, 33, 34–35

Alcohol, 51, 98, 178

Allergies, 74, 79, 102, 108, 120

ALS (amyotrophic lateral sclerosis), 37, 39, 40–41

Alzheimer's disease (AD), 37, 65, 67, 100, 199

Amnesia, 67

Anemia, 43, 45, 46

Angina, 183, 184

Anti-inflammatories, 37, 46, 80–81, 139–42, 209

Antioxidants, 15, 27, 33, 37, 93, 200, 209

Anxiety, 97–102, 141, 179

Aphrodisiac, 50

Arteriosclerosis, 3, 80–81, 201

Arthritis, 37

Ash colored fleabane, 157

– B –

Asthma, 60, 73–77, 133

Astralagus root, 45

Atopic dermatitis, 43

Atractylodes rhizome, 45

Attention deficit disorder (ADD), 68

Autoimmune disorders, 32

Beta-carotene, 32

Bifidobacteria, 61

Biphenols, 99

Bitter melon, 171, 173

Blindness, 31

Blood
    clots, 183–87
    lipid levels, 164, 169
    pressure, 188, 201–6
    sugar, 164, 167, 171–74, 177, 195

Blood-brain barrier (BBB), 32, 33, 110

Boswellia, 131

Bronchitis, 79, 81–82

Bupleurum root, 58

– C –

Cancer, 37, 47, 55, 59, 178
    breast, 14, 19, 203, 205

cervix, 89

colon, 14, 21, 44, 203, 205, 209

kidney, 59

lung, 19, 21, 89

mouth, 21, 89

ovary, 19, 21

prevention, 31

risk, 32

skin, 10–12, 25-27

statistics, 1–2

stomach, 14

treatment booster, 113

treatments, 3–27

Carotenoids, 32

Carpal tunnel syndrome, 82

Cataracts, 33, 34, 35

Chanca piedra, 171, 172, 173

Charcoal, 149

Chemotherapy, 5, 7, 16, 17, 43, 45, 47

Cholesterol
    HDL, 196–97
    high, 32, 35, 46, 164, 167, 169, 195–200, 207–10
    LDL, 32, 164, 167, 196–97, 208–10

Chronic fatigue syndrome, 43, 188, 190–91

Chuangxiong, 45

Meadowsweet, 148–49

Menopause, 55, 122, 197

Migraines, 117-25, 188, 190

Moles, 12

Multiple sclerosis (MS), 32, 118

Musk mallow, 131

– N –

Natto, 183, 184, 186, 187–90, 193–94

Natural killer cells, 43, 89

Neem, 171

Neurodegenerative disease, 32

Nopal cactus, 167

NSAIDs (non-steroidal anti-inflammatory drugs), 127, 139, 141–42, 209

– O –

Obesity, 161, 167, 178, 179

Orthostatic hypotension, 60

Osteoperosis, 187, 194

– P –

Panax ginseng, 46, 189

Parkinson's disease, 32, 37, 100, 110, 118

Pasanabheda, 157

Pata de vaca, 171–72

Pau d'arco, 22

Pedra hume caa, 171, 172–73

Peony root, 46

Phytochemicals, 21, 22

Pinellia tuber, 58

Plaque, arterial, 80–81

Pneumonia, 61–62

Polysaccharides, 4, 13

Preneoplastic lesions, 59

Probiotics, 61, 122

Psoriasis, 12, 79, 88

– R –

Radiation, 43

Rehmannia root, 46

Rheumatoid arthritis (RA), 27, 37, 38, 43, 79, 127–31

Rhubarb, 149

Rough chaff tree, 157

– S –

Sarcoma, 20, 22, 47

Scutellaria root, 58

Sedge, 157

Selenium, 15

Serotonin, 110

Shark cartilage, 16, 203–4

Shilapushpa, 157

Shingles, 26, 103, 106, 107

Skin cancer, 10–12, 25–27

Sleeplessness, 100

Smoking, 34

Snake bites, 20–21, 22

Spleen cells, 43

Statin drugs, 195, 198, 207, 210, 211

Stevia, 171, 173

Stroke, 110, 113, 117, 183, 184, 201

– T –

T-cells, 4, 43–44, 88, 89

Taxol®, 19, 22

Tonsillitis, 60

Transient ischemic attacks (TIAs), 189

Tumor Necrosis Factor (TNF), 4, 89

Tumors, 5, 44, 59, 90

– U –

Ulcerative colitis, 43, 79, 118, 133–38

Ulcers, 20–21, 22, 46, 61, 139, 140, 149

Umbrella's edge, 157

Urinary tract infections, 151–58

Uveitis, 79

– V –

Varicose veins, 82, 83, 188

Vitamin E, 32, 88

– X –

Xanthophylls, 33

Get the underground cures of tomorrow—today! And be among the first to know!

This book is based on the research and discoveries of the Health Sciences Institute (HSI). HSI is a unique members-only organization, built upon a vast network of doctors and researchers from around the world, that's dedicated to doing one thing: breaking the barriers that big-money medicine has placed before revolutionary natural cures—and bringing those cures to you *right now*!

Unlike anything before it, HSI doesn't represent the opinion of a single, self-appointed "guru," but it contains the unmatched combined wisdom of the world's most formidable medical minds.

Through the monthly HSI *Members Alert* newsletter, regular email updates, and online Forum discussions, we inform our members about exciting new breakthroughs in natural healing, show them how to use them, what results to expect, and where to get them.

The clear and easy-to-read HSI *Members Alert* has become a legend in the alternative medical industry as a quintessential source for cutting-edge medical discoveries. Many physicians all over the world use the *Members Alert* to bring their own patients medical solutions and treatments available nowhere else—including the underground cures you've read about in this book.

Hundreds of members have thanked us for bringing them the newest solutions that work where other therapies—mainstream and alternative—have failed.

- *"I cannot thank HSI enough for helping my daughter eliminate her unrelenting bought with psoriasis. Because of you, the Lovelands have a lot to be thankful for this Thanksgiving. Best Wishes."* G. Loveland.

- *"My health has really improved over the last several months. I get a lot of brand-new, cutting-edge information from you that cannot be found easily anywhere else." Bob A.*

• *"Every day we fervently thank God for guiding me to choose [the therapy HSI featured] to treat my husband's liver cancer. From the day of his first dose, he began improving almost overnight. Now, he's completely tumor free!" Jocelyn Webb, Pryor, OK*

Now, you can continue to get the latest breakthrough cures for everything from arthritis, to cancer, to heart disease, and more by joining the Health Sciences Institute today. As a member of HSI, you'll have the opportunity to take advantage of exclusive special reports, first access to hard-to-get products and services, access to a worldwide network of doctors and researchers, and much more.

Simply return the New Member Certificate below, along with your first annual membership payment of $49 to activate your membership, which includes 12 monthly issues of the HSI *Members Alert* newsletter and all the benefits described above. Reply today!

(Cut along dotted line and return to HSI, P.O. Box 925, Frederick, MD 21705-9913)

New Membership Certificate

❏ **YES!** I would like to join the Health Sciences Institute for the low price of $49 today. That includes 12 issues of the HSI *Members Alert*, which I can cancel at any time for a full refund of all unmailed issues.

Name:_____

Address:_____

City:_____ State:_____ Zip:_____

Phone: (_____)_____

E-mail: _____
(To receive your FREE health updates.)

❏ My check is enclosed for $ _____ made payable to Health Sciences Institute
(Maryland residents add 5% sales tax)

❏ Please charge my: ❏ Visa ❏ MasterCard ❏ American Express ❏ Discover

Card #:_____ Expires:_____

Signature:_____

PHSIBC01

Return this reply to: Health Sciences Institute
PO Box 925 • Frederick, MD 21705-9913
(or fax to: 410-230-1273)
www.HSIBaltimore.com

New breakthroughs and urgent health news sent directly to you ABSOLUTELY FREE!

Be among the first to benefit from all-natural cures and life-extending discoveries that the rest of the world won't know about for another generation—or longer. Best of all…it's <u>absolutely FREE</u>—no strings attached.

Now you can receive the Health Sciences Institute's exclusive e-Alerts, normally sent only to its members. Using the power of the internet, HSI is able to share their breaking discoveries and insights <u>as they happen</u>. And now you can receive them—FREE.

Each day, HSI receives hundreds of e-mails from members. Here are just a few examples:

- *Boris S. wrote, "Thank you again for your updates and alerts. You have been consistent and perfect," following our story on the food industry's attempt to introduce natural bacteria killers.*

- *Ruth W. wrote to say, "What a wonderful report on NIH ignoring the true cause(s) of disease," after reading our alert about NIH's decision to lower standards for high cholesterol, in turn recommending drugs for millions more Americans.*

- *And Dr. Fritz writes: "Your e-mails, just as your newsletter, are most important for me. Thank you for what you are doing for your members."*

Signing up is simple. If you are already a member of HSI, just send a blank e-mail to hsi_sub@agoramail.net. If you are not a member, send a blank e-mail to nonhsi_sub@agoramail.net.

(We share your concerns over privacy. HSI will never sell your e-mail address. And, of course, you can unsubscribe at any time.)

Sign up for **FREE** today!

STRONGER THAN STEROIDS
Get cortisone-like relief in as little as a week...
All-natural breakthrough leaves old standbys in the dust...

Natalie Collins couldn't even crawl into bed without hurting. It hurt when she sat. It hurt when she walked. It just plain hurt all the time. And nothing would help. As she told us:

"Ibuprofen turned the fire down a notch or two for awhile. But within a few weeks, I couldn't even notice the difference...

"The only thing that helped were the cortisone shots. And I'm scared stiff to repeat them because of the side effects..."

And then Natalie tried something that beat them all—with no side effects.

"I was feeling better in less than a week. I haven't felt this good in years. I can stand up all day on the job. And the best part is I can keep taking this every day. Plus, I just keep on feeling better and better every week."

Flexanol—the most complete joint formula.

Natalie's transformation wasn't a fluke. Flexanol literally delivers 10 times more joint support than the old standbys.*

The life restoring miracle of MSM

MSM (Methyl-sulfonyl-methane) is the miracle molecule that supplies our bodies with sulfur, the fourth most abundant mineral in human tissue. And it turns out to be absolutely critical to healthy joints because we rely on sulfur to create and regenerate all of our cells.

According to Dr. Ronald M. Lawrence, Assistant Clinical Prof. of the UCLA School of Medicine and Founding Member of the American Association for the Study of Pain—people with arthritis often lack the proper amount of sulfur to let the body heal itself.

Dr. Lawrence recently completed a double blind study to test the effectiveness of MSM on pain relief in arthritic patients. 80% of the patients felt most of their pain vanish.

MSM speeds nutrients to the sites of tissue damage, helps the body get rid of pain causing toxins, helps regenerate healthy new cells, and even repairs damaged cartilage...And best of all, MSM is literally as safe as water!

That's the result of 30 years of research at the Oregon Health Science University in Portland, Oregon. In three decades, they uncovered no side effects. And just like Natalie Rollins, most of the patients in the Oregon study reported improvement within a week!

Sound good so far? It gets better. Because Flexanol brings together every major joint support breakthrough of the last 30 years. Starting, of course, with:

Glucosamine HCL—To help rebuild damaged cartilage and improve flexibility

Unlike NSAIDs and steroid treatments, Flexanol's power actually increases with repeated use. Glucosamine HCL is a big reason why. You may feel it 'kick in' after a number of weeks, adding to the good work that began with the MSM.

Nine clinical studies now prove that supplementing with glucosamine can turn things around and then some. More than 1,500 patients who took glucosamine daily for 4 weeks found that it restored joint flexibility, reversed joint damage, and helped repair cartilage...all without side effects.

Sea Cucumber—A fabulous natural source of the joint protector Chondroitin

This relative of the starfish hails from the waters of Australia's Great Barrier Reef. And it's so astonishingly effective, that the Australian government has actually designated it as an official arthritis treatment!

Sea cucumber can pack a powerful 'one-two punch' against joint pain because it contains two important compounds: natural chondroitin and more glucosamine. Together, this combo is just what you need to 'jump start' healthy new cartilage.

EPA and DHA—To root out the causes of painful inflammation

Next, Flexanol goes to work on the inflammation that swells joints and adds to your pain. It does so with EPA and DHA. Both are substances that occur naturally in your body, called Omega-3 fatty acids. Several studies show that Omega-3 fatty acids don't

* Flexanol includes 10 proven joint supportive nutrients where most products include only one.

just mask inflammation, but actually stop the autoimmune reactions that cause it.

In fact, studies have shown that patients who take these fatty acids were able to reduce or discontinue their doses of NSAIDs. Just imagine feeling better without the painkillers than you did with them!

Boswellia—To stop pain before it begins

Natural healers in India have been using boswellia serrata for centuries and it may be the most amazing pain reliever in all of nature. Modern researchers even go so far as to say:

"The therapeutic action of [boswellia] includes: reduction of joint swelling, restoration and improvement of blood supply to inflamed joints, pain relief, increased mobility, amelioration of morning stiffness, steroid-sparing effects and general improvement in the quality of life."—James Braly, MD

Plus, by slowing down the leukotriene cycle—a very important cause of inflammation—boswellia helps stop inflammation before it starts! And it works for nearly everyone.

In a double blind clinical trial of 175 people, 97% reported relief of arthritis symptoms. No one complained of any undesirable side effects.

Borage Oil—Proven in a definitive university study to shrink swollen joints

Borage oil has long been a trusted joint healer in Europe. And scientists now know exactly why. It turns out to be a terrific natural source of the Omega-6 fatty acid GLA (gamma-linolenic acid).

A year-long study at the University of Massachusetts Medical Center now shows that patients taking GLA may be 6 times more likely to have dramatic improvement in joint pain and joint swelling compared to patients taking a placebo.

Ginger—The Caribbean secret for relief

You probably knew that ginger root is one of the all-time great healing herbs, prized for centuries by natural healers from China to India and even ancient Greece.

Caribbean islanders know another terrific secret about it. For years, they've used ginger root to treat arthritis pain and inflammation. And research shows it works! How? By increasing the circulation while actually reducing inflammation.

Each of the above by itself has been shown to help relieve pain, but the real miracle happens when you put them all together with other supporting vitamins and minerals. The synergy does what no other single supplement can do.

Famed nutritional authority praises Flexanol as STATE OF THE ART

"Flexanol goes well beyond virtually all nutriceutical formulas in its comprehensiveness towards helping the body overcome the many discomforts of arthritis. All of its ingredients carry both scientific and anecdotal support for the formula's success. Flexanol contains more generous amounts of scientifically supported ingredients than other formulas I have seen in the recent past. Congratulations on making Flexanol..."—Dr. Arnold J. Susser, R.P., Ph.D. President, Nutrition Society of America.

Send for your RISK-FREE supply today.

Flexanol is 100% natural and side-effect free! It has been rigorously tested for quality, purity and potency and each bottle is stamped with an expiration date to ensure freshness.

We promise you can feel better IN A WEEK—OR LESS!

You'll get out of bed without wincing...bend, kneel and walk through your day without pain...feel life returning to your joints...and it all starts within the first 7 days! Then, week after week, you'll feel more free to do what you want. Not only will those stiff joints unlock, but your range of motion will be restored. So you can...reclaim the active life you deserve!

It's happened already for so many people. And it will happen for you. Or simply return the unused portion within 60 days and we'll cheerfully refund your purchase price—in full.

So why not try Flexanol right now—completely RISK-FREE...and think of the free, active lifestyle you stand to regain. Don't delay. Let us hear from you today. A 1-month supply of Flexanol is just $34.95 (plus $4.50 s/h) or, save on 3 months for $94.85 (plus $4.50 s/h) or 6 months for $189.70 (FREE s/h).

Call NorthStar Nutritionals at: 1-800-311-1950, ORDER CODE FLEX
(or, 203-699-4438).
Send checks to NorthStar Nutritionals,
Dept. FLEX, P.O. Box 925,
Frederick, MD 21705.

Patients with shellfish allergies should not take Flexanol.

This statement has not been evaluated by the Food and Drug Administration. This product is not intended to diagnose, treat, cure, or prevent any disease.

228

Order Form

To order any of the books in the **How to Fight Series** simply check the title(s) of the book(s) you want, fill in the number of copies you wish to order, add in the appropriate amount of shipping and handling (see box below), and mail in this completed form.

❑ **How to Fight Cancer & Win** ___ copy/copies at **$19.95** ea. $_____
[680SFCBK]

❑ **How to Fight Prostate Cancer & Win** ___ copy/copies at **$19.95** ea. $_____
[680SBPRO]

❑ **How to Fight Arthritis & Win** ___ copy/copies at **$19.95** ea. $_____
[680SHFA]

❑ **How to Fight Heart Disease & Win** ___ copy/copies at **$19.95** ea. $_____
[680SFHD]

Shipping and Handling
1-3 books add $5.00 S&H
4-9 books add $10.00 S&H
10+ books add $15.00 S&H

SUBTOTAL: $_____

SHIPPING & HANDLING: $_____
(see S&H box for details)

TOTAL: $_____

Check method of payment: *(All orders processed in US dollars.)*

❑ My check is enclosed for $ _____ made payable to **Agora Health Books**.
(Maryland residents add 5% sales tax)

❑ Please charge my: ❑ Visa ❑ MasterCard ❑ American Express ❑ Discover

Card #:_____ Expires: _____

Signature: _____

Ship to:

Name: _____

Address: _____

City:_____ State:_____ Zip: _____

Phone: (_____) _____
(In case we have a question about your order)

e-mail: _____
(To receive FREE health e-Alerts)

Mail in your order today!
Agora Health Books • PO Box 977 • Dept. M680AHB • Frederick, MD 21705-9838
Visit us at www.agorahealthbooks.com

For fastest service call 1-888-821-3609 and ask for code M680AHB
or fax your credit card order to 1-410-230-1273

M680AHB

PRO-1

Notes